Three Levels for S... ...g,
Posture, and Fitness
in Just 10 Minutes a Day

28 DAYS

OF

CHAIR EXERCISES

FOR WEIGHT LOSS

99 ILLUSTRATED EXERCISES
ORGANIZED INTO 28 ROUTINES

Ottie Oz

Disclaimer Notice:

Please note that the information contained within this document is for educational and entertainment purposes only. All effort has been expended to present accurate, up-to-date, reliable, complete information. No warranties of any kind are declared or implied. Readers acknowledge that the author is not engaged in the rendering of legal, financial, medical, or professional advice. The content within this book has been derived from various sources. Please consult a licensed professional before attempting any techniques outlined in this book. By reading this document, the reader agrees that under no circumstances are the authors responsible for any losses, direct or indirect, which are incurred as a result of the use of the information contained within this document, including, but not limited to, errors, omissions, or inaccuracies.

Not all exercises suit everyone, and this or any other exercise program may result in injury. Please consult your doctor before beginning this or any other exercise program, especially if you have any chronic or recurring condition or are pregnant, nursing, or elderly. This exercise program is not recommended if you experience chest pains, have uncontrolled blood pressure, or have other chronic diseases. By performing any of the exercises in this program, you assume all risks of injury from doing so. The authors are not responsible or liable for any injury or loss you may sustain by participating in this exercise program. Always warm up before beginning any workout, and never exercise beyond the level you feel comfortable with. Please stop exercising immediately if you experience pain, soreness, fatigue, shortness of breath, dizziness, light-headedness, blurred vision, headache, nausea, sickness, illness, dehydration, excessive sweating, or any other discomfort. If any of these symptoms persist after you stop exercising, please seek medical help immediately. This exercise program and instructions provided in this program are not intended and should not be used as a substitute for professional medical advice, diagnosis, or treatment. The authors make no representation or warranty, whether express or implied, concerning the safety, usefulness, or result of this exercise program.

Table of Contents

Discover our Exclusive Joint & Ankle Sequences!

Scan QR code or go on

http://chairexercises.littlegeckopublishing.com

Elevate your mobility and ease discomfort with our expertly designed sequences. Perfect for enhancing flexibility, reducing pain, or adding mindfulness to your day, these sequences are the ultimate upgrade to your wellness routine. Start feeling the difference today!

Introduction

How old would you be if you didn't know how old you are?
— Reverend Clarence H. Wilson

We are living in an ever-changing world, and one positive change seen in recent times is the level of interest in longevity. There is also increasing interest in the mature population regarding leading a physically healthier life into the later years of life.

Recent population figures indicate that there are over 750 million people alive today over the age of 65 (United Nations, 2022) , more than at any other time in recorded history. To put this into context, this is nearly six times higher than in 1950. During this same period, the world's life expectancy has also risen sharply. In 1950, globally, the average person was expected to live 47 years. Today, this figure sits at 71 years (Dattani et al., 2023). Someone born 70 years ago will have been born shortly after the Second World War—before telephones and even televisions were in every home, before man walked on the moon, before computers and the internet became mainstream, and before mobile phones were even an idea. By the opposite measure, someone born today will almost certainly live to see the new century—2100.

The rise in life expectancy and the number of older adults still with us can be attributed to many reasons, one of which is how many more of us are leading relatively active lifestyles. For many seniors, living an active lifestyle is not necessarily something new. They, after all, grew up in a time when children would generally spend their free time playing outside rather than inside.If you are fortunate enough to have lived to a great age, what may have changed since these years is the ease with which you are able to execute these physical activities. For some, the struggles might be limited to specific body parts and activities. For others, it may even be more severe and interfere with everyday life, like getting out of bed or keeping balance while on their feet.

With advances in the understanding of the human body and ways in which we can treat aging muscles and body parts, the increasingly difficult future many older citizens face (especially with regard to the feeling of the body failing them) need not be your future. What if this future can be avoided by simply using an everyday item that is probably already in your possession and that you already use every day?

In this book, we will explore how the simple four-legged chair can be used to turn back your body's clock. Through targeted exercises, you will soon rebuild withering muscles, restore balance, and slowly but surely gain confidence, leading to an improved quality of life. We will also look into the benefits of remaining active as you age, provide a step-by-step guide as to how to execute chair exercises, assist you in building and maintaining your exercise plan and routine, address weight management, and ultimately leave you leading your best life possible.

Being Active and Embracing Fitness at Any Age

Those who think they have not time for bodily exercise
will sooner or later have to find time for illness.
— Edward Stanley

As alluded to earlier, the portion of the population living into their 60s and beyond has never been greater. It is one thing to be alive at that age, and it is a completely different take if you are still able to live life during these years. For many, to continue living life and enjoying everything they hold dear, it is of great importance that people look after their physical well-being as their bodies morph.

Before we delve deeper into the topic, it's so good to see the significant impact of exercise on older individuals. It's not uncommon to see people in their 60s, 70s, and even 80s achieving incredible physical activity results. For instance, within the running clubs, numerous members actively participate in marathons and ultramarathons in their later years. Or they are playing tennis with friends. This challenges common perceptions, proving that an active lifestyle is more than just for the younger generation. It's very pleasing to see the older population being active—taking up sports they had never done before and excelling at them! These examples are powerful testaments to the possibilities that await when one embraces an active lifestyle, regardless of age. I'm sure you've heard that before that age; it's just a number, right? People have varying levels of mobility, but fortunately, you can easily modify exercises to suit individual needs. You can perform many of them while sitting and still reap the benefits.

While not every senior is destined to perform extreme feats at the age groups mentioned above, it is no longer uncommon to see them taking part in physical activities like surfing or squash weekly with people half their age or even newsworthy when folks in their 70s summit great mountain peaks. These active lifestyles continue to play a significant role in the changing face of mature people.

No longer is it considered the norm for seniors to spend the day alternating between the bed, the couch, and the seat on the porch, with their bodies slowly shriveling and muscles and tendons wasting away. Sure, not many are as spry as they once were, but no physical activity (or attempts at it) should be discounted. Not only that, but it is now commonplace to see an older person leading an independent lifestyle.

Being able to maintain these lifestyles is but one benefit of regular physical activity and exercise. Tying into the topic of longevity and more active lifestyles, research has also shown the medical benefits of regular physical activity. Studies have specifically focused on the role that active lifestyles play in lowering the chances of contracting heart diseases, diabetes, strokes, and many forms of cancer (World Health Organization, 2018). These diseases are also among the leading causes of death throughout the world, so one can see how increased levels of physical activity across the population have likely led to people living longer lives.

Over the years, a number of studies have also focused on the positive mental benefits of physical activity. One such recent study showed that the risk of depression among older adults, whether they had chronic pain or not, was lower when they performed moderate physical activity regularly (Laird et al., 2023). This specific study included those who already suffer from chronic pain in order to eliminate criticism of bias in previous studies (where healthier individuals made up the observed subjects).

It has furthermore been illustrated how physical activity in the elderly unlocks key benefits when it comes to movement and improved cognitive function (better command of one's own body, such as factors relating to strength and flexibility). The same study also saw improved concentration and more focused relaxation (Picorelli et al., 2014).

There are, of course, many rollover benefits as well, like social benefits. For example, a golfer who is able to remain active within his society will be able to maintain his long-standing friendships a lot better should he remain capable of meeting his golfing friends weekly for a round and enjoying a drink thereafter.

The U.S. Department of Health and Human Services (2018) lists many more benefits of regular physical activity: improved sleep, reduced levels of anxiety, and reduced blood pressure in the short term. In addition to the abovementioned benefits, in the long term, the following benefits are listed: balance and coordination (important for avoiding falls), improved bone health, and healthier weight management (which we will explore in depth in a later chapter).

Suppose you have time to go through the source material for many of the studies mentioned above. In that case, it will become clear that they do not necessarily always list what physical activity was done. You, as someone to whom chair exercises are clearly a topic of interest, may then be left wondering if any of the above applies to chair exercises. The good news is that they are.

Owing to their versatile nature, chair exercises indeed hold many benefits. Some of these include the following:

- **Convenience:** It can be done anywhere and at any time.
- **Inclusivity:** Anyone who is able to sit upright under their own power will be able to do chair exercises.
- **Muscle building:** This is not just limited to the arms but rather the entire body.
- **Cardio workouts are possible:** There are truly exercises that target a variety of facets of physical health.
- **Improved mobility:** Perhaps this is what many will be most familiar with (when picturing rehabilitation patients).

Now that we've looked through some of the benefits of physical activity and chair exercises specifically, it is also important that we examine some of the common misconceptions and false narratives surrounding the older population and exercise. The foremost of these is the most frequent excuse: "I am too old" (or a variation thereof). There are endless examples of amazing elderly folks doing amazing things. You only need to head over to the Guinness World Records website and type "oldest" in the search bar to find some of these (from the oldest active mechanic to the oldest person to perform a headstand).

Having previously been an easy escape route, the claims that all exercise worsens current physical ailments (such as arthritis) have been studied in depth and debunked through numerous undertakings. The Mayo Clinic (2023) even explicitly prescribes exercise as an essential tool in fighting arthritis, citing range of motion, strengthening, and aerobic exercises as key.

How often through our lives have we heard elder relatives or friends state that they are too limited in what they can do? From not being able to stand for extended periods to having limited mobility, these are not excuses that can be generally used for chair exercises. The exercises in this book are crafted to accommodate a wide range of situations. Bundled under this branch of excuses, many of us are of the belief that our risk of falling increases if we take part in physical activities. While this might hold some truth for activities that involve standing, chair exercises, for the most part, eliminate this aspect.

Lastly, there's the excuse that just about every person has used at least once in their life: "I don't have time." This is a simple case of finding your *why*, a topic to which we have dedicated an entire chapter in this book. Without your *why*, it is highly unlikely that your exercise program will be sustainable. This will, of course, vary from person to person, but the importance remains. "I don't have enough time" only applies if your grander goals are not a priority.

Now that we have had a look at some of the benefits and challenges that many face, we can dive into some other aspects. Exercise is a good launching pad, but to successfully achieve an improved quality of life, it needs to be coupled with a smarter diet and, better yet, weight management.

Managing Weight Loss with Exercises and Savvy Food Choices

Exercise is king. Nutrition is queen.
Put them together and you've got a kingdom.

— Jack Lalanne

"Lose 20 pounds in 3 weeks" is how a typical infomercial starts, making promise after promise on the benefits of their new "miracle" product, which will apparently leave you looking and feeling younger than ever before. Now and again, they will even feature a so-called expert or have a celebrity (or pseudo-celebrity) endorse the product. Have you ever wondered why these infomercials rarely, if ever, feature anyone with a Ph.D. or Dr. in their title? This is no coincidence, as a doctor is required to take a Hippocratic oath, and should they knowingly mete out bad advice or suggest treatments not based on and rooted in medical science, there is a good chance they'll never be able to practice again.

What happens to the aforementioned experts or celebrities if the product is found to not yield all the benefits promised? Nothing. What many of these miracle products fail to mention is that behind the scenes, all those who consumed the product were more than likely also put on an exercise program as well as an adjusted and controlled eating plan. Imagine the world we could be living in if regular exercise and healthier eating plans were pushed to the front and center of the public psyche.

This book follows the approach that calls for a combination of both exercises and a healthy diet to create what is called a calorie deficit for weight loss (or maintenance). The concept of calorie deficits is very simple: Is your body using everything you put into it? If you eat and drink more calories than you use throughout a given day, you'll have a calorie surplus. A sustained surplus will result in weight gain, while a sustained deficit over time will result in weight loss. On the whole, small differences should balance out in the long term.

It is also of utmost importance that we start by acknowledging that, in order to continue functioning optimally, the body does actually need calories. So it goes without saying that you should not deprive yourself of food or drink. We will just be seeking to eat and drink in a healthier manner and in the quantities we need. When you exercise more, you will require additional calories. The converse holds true when you move less.

These required quantities vary based on a broad number of factors. The best estimates have the average adult male requiring 2,500 kcal, while the average female requires 2,000 kcal daily (NHS, 2021). Some factors alluded to earlier that cause variations in requirements include age, weight, height, and how much exercise the individual does. For individuals 51 years of age and older, it is estimated that this figure could range between 2,000 and 2,800 kcal for males and between 1,600 and 2,200 kcal for females (Callahan et al., 2020). And yet again, I want to reiterate that it depends on the person and their circumstances.

There are two important factors I would like to point out before we continue. Firstly, as with most long-term and sustainable lifestyle changes, you will not be expected to go cold turkey and immediately and completely overhaul your diet. And secondly, while the subject of calorie reduction can sound overly scientific and complicated, it definitely need not be. Sure, there are definitely more precise ways of determining the number of calories you need. And yes, there are definitely more scientific ways to go about logging how many calories you consume daily. However, many find that lifestyle changes fail when the person feels like it becomes a chore to keep it going, which would be the case if it involves frequent and overcomplicated calculations.

We are therefore looking at easier and more practical ways in which we can avoid this. And, thankfully, there are means available. You could think of it in terms of an artistic interpretation of a tree by two artists. One artist might use a fine paintbrush and intricately and meticulously paint each branch and leaf of the tree. Another might use a broader brush and simply paint the brown base of the tree and a green circle on top. From a few feet away, most people will easily be able to identify the latter as a tree, despite the lack of care taken in producing the painting.

The same goes for how we will approach the concept of creating a calorie deficit. Let's not focus on day-to-day calorie counting but rather on creating the best possible overall picture with our available means. There are many natural and easy ways of reducing calories, and the simplest way of doing this is to create a healthier eating plan containing more whole foods.

What exactly are whole foods? While there are no strict accreditations or certificates that are issued identifying them, whole and unprocessed foods are foods that are sold as close as possible to their natural state. The next time you're at the grocery store, you should be easily able to identify them. They are commonly unpackaged (or minimally packaged) and free of additives. Unfortunately, there has been a great drive toward convenience over the past few decades, to the point where many associate whole foods with blandness. Again, this is certainly not the case, as spices and healthier condiments form part of cleaner diets.

So, what exactly does a healthy and balanced diet look like? In keeping with the latest scientific medical findings, the USDA (2020) recommends the following (with some examples listed):

- Consume more whole and unprocessed fruits and vegetables (rich in vitamins, fiber, antioxidants, potassium, manganese, iron, etc.):
  - apples
  - bananas
  - oranges
  - blueberries
  - strawberries
  - avocado
  - broccoli
  - carrots
  - kale

- Consume more whole grains (loaded with carbohydrates and fiber):
  - steel-cut oats
  - brown rice
  - quinoa
  - whole wheat pasta and wraps
  - certain breads (e.g., Ezekiel bread) in moderation

- Consume more lean meats and pulses (high in protein):
  - eggs
  - lean beef
  - chicken breasts
  - salmon
  - tuna
  - lentils
  - chickpeas
  - beans

- Include healthy oils (for healthy fats):
  - olive oil
  - canola oil

- Include dairy (the less processed, the better):
  - low-fat milk
  - cheese
  - yogurt

While not outwardly encouraged, the occasional consumption of processed foods and drinks does not necessarily cancel out all progress. Simply try as far as possible to hop back onto the wagon as soon as possible. It should also be noted that there are varying degrees of food processing. It is advisable to avoid the most processed products (referred to as ultra-processed). Some common examples of ultra-processed foods include mass-produced bread, most mass-produced cereals, chips, most carbonated drinks, yogurts with fruit flavoring, and mass-produced meats.

So, what are some of the changes we can look to implement? Firstly, perhaps rethink the manner in which you consume food. Combining foods into a solitary dish is nothing new. Dishes like curries and stews have been around for millennia and can pretty much be found across every continent and in every culture. For the purpose of adding fruits and vegetables to your diet, why not consider having more homemade smoothies in summer and soups in winter? Consider using wraps instead of bread, honey instead of sugar, iced tea instead of carbonated drinks, oats instead of cornflakes, and chicken breasts and lean beef or pork steak cuts instead of chicken and beef burgers, sausages, and ham. While it might seem difficult to navigate at first, you'll soon pick it up.

By now, many of you will already be wondering, *How do I know how big a portion is?* While these are obviously not scientifically accurate to a tee, there are a few simple unofficial rules of thumb you can use as a cheat sheet to get an idea of portion sizes:

- **Open palm:** One portion of meats and other proteins
- **Closed fist:** One portion of fruits and vegetables
- **Cupped palm:** One portion of grains (and other carbohydrates)
- **Thumb:** One portion of oils (and other fats)

By replacing the heavily processed foods you may currently be consuming with more of the above, you are already creating a calorie deficit relative to your current status quo. By adding regular exercise to the equation, the benefits multiply. To further illustrate the effect of exercise on the body's use of calories, consider roughly how much you need to exercise to "cancel out" the following commonly consumed goods:

- 1 can of soda equals 26 minutes of walking or 13 minutes of running.
- 1 standard chocolate bar equals 42 minutes of walking or 22 minutes of running.

- 1 standard bag of chips equals 31 minutes of walking or 16 minutes of running.
- 1 iced cinnamon bun equals 1 hour and 17 minutes of walking or 40 minutes of running.

It's not advisable to adopt an attitude where you bargain with yourself—like drinking a can of soda with the justification of walking the dog later. This approach rarely works. I echo Dr. Yoni Freedhoff's sentiment that you can't outrun your fork. I've tried it myself and failed a few times. A balanced approach is key: both exercise and a healthy diet need to become integral parts of your life.

The final point of discussion in this chapter pertains to whether or not chair exercises can effectively be used for weight loss. The simple answer is yes. As long as you are using up energy and burning more calories (which you do even by simply moving or even more so when exercising at a high intensity) than what you have consumed, you will be able to lose weight. This obviously differs from person to person, but in any event, you are definitely better off doing some exercises than none at all.

Hopefully, you have a better understanding by now of the principles of weight loss and management. In the end, it is as simple as asking yourself, "Am I using more calories than I'm putting into my body?" If yes, you will create a calorie deficit. Sustain this over a period of time, and you should notice weight loss.

Finding Your Why, Committing to New Routines, And Achieving Your Fitness Goals

He who has a why to live can bear almost any how.
— Friedrich Nietzsche

Many diets fail. Understanding why they do can be a key in our journey toward a healthier lifestyle. The reasons for these failures often come down to a few missteps. One major pitfall is setting unrealistic goals or not setting them at all. Getting caught up in ambitious targets that are not feasible in the short term is easy. Another common issue is focusing excessively on calorie counting. This can lead to an unhealthy obsession rather than a balanced approach to eating.

However, the most significant oversight is failing to recognize that adopting a healthier lifestyle is a long-term commitment. It involves gradually and consistently replacing unhealthy habits with healthier ones—creating new routines. This isn't just about a temporary change in diet; it's about embarking on a journey to discover what works best for you personally, understanding that this process takes time and patience.

Finding your "why" is a crucial part of this journey. I learned it the hard way. Like many, I couldn't wrap my head around a healthy lifestyle for quite a long time. I found myself trying different diets; some of them were strict ones. I was "on a diet" very often. It was almost "my thing." Admittedly, they have offered short-term solutions but never lasted long enough if I managed to get through them. You might assume that after more than several failed attempts, I would realize something is wrong and that these diets don't' really work. Yet, it took me long and painful years to realize this approach wasn't practical or effective.

My good friend's journey to a healthier lifestyle was inspiring and surprising. We used to be very active kids—constantly on the move. The afternoons were spent playing volleyball with classmates and neighborhood kids. Summer holidays were filled with endless bike rides and swims in the lake. As time went on, our paths crossed less and less.

While I was increasingly engrossed in music school and spent most of my time in classes and doing homework, she explored different passions. She had a knack for languages. She spent most of her time buried in books and taking part in language clubs. This intellectual pursuit, though enriching, meant less time for physical activities for both of us. The active lifestyle of our childhood slowly faded into the background. Our diet, increasingly distant from any notion of healthiness, followed suit.

As time passed, we transformed from wide-eyed kids into all-knowing teenagers—in our minds, the masters of the universe. And then it arrived—exams, school graduation, university applications.

We've been accepted at different universities in separate towns, yet we stayed connected. Despite our busy academic lives, we met roughly every six months. The first time I saw her after we parted ways, I was taken aback. She lost a significant amount of weight. She said that she had joined a weight loss club and followed a strict diet for six weeks. However, during our day together, I couldn't help but notice her indulgence in sugary treats—a diet I couldn't help thinking, with a touch of irony, that I could get on board with.

The next time we met, she appeared different from just half a year before. She was devastated that she had regained the weight she lost and added more. This cycle continued for a few years. Our meetings became less frequent, but she dropped a bombshell during one of our phone conversations—she was training for a half-marathon. The news was more than surprising; it was astounding.

I attended her first event, as I wanted to be there for her.

I couldn't wait to hear what had happened. A half-marathon?! She shared her turning point with me when we sat down to catch up. After one particularly disheartening episode with junk food, she felt a physical and emotional low. She hit the bottom with her dieting. She realized that she wanted a change—a lasting change.

She started with simple walks. They challenged her more than expected. But instead of discouraging her, these difficulties fueled her determination.

Slowly, her short walks turned into longer ones, taking shapes as short runs and, eventually, long-distance running. She confided that her mindset had shifted: it was no longer about restricting herself but about nourishing her body and mind with healthy food to support her new passion. She had accidentally stumbled upon her "why," and it was running. To be able to train and take part in all sorts of running competitions, she had to take care of her body.

As I listened to her story, I felt a surge of happiness for her. I did. She had found her purpose, her motivation—her "why." And as for me, I realized I was still on my journey, searching for my own.

That first half-marathon was a milestone. She may not have set a record, but her personal accomplishment was immense. She had found her "why."

I am well aware that this is an example of extreme proportions, but it can be applied to any situation and any *why*. There are limitless examples, and they will almost certainly differ from person to person. For many, the reasoning for wanting to stay healthy might be as simple as living to see and play with their grandchildren. It may be to remain fit enough to continue playing a sport they enjoy participating in. It may be for more personal reasons, like remaining confident in their movements or even remaining confident in their appearance.

As much as there is no one-size-fits-all for finding your *why*, there is also no single approach that will guarantee your successful journey to a healthier you. For each person, this journey will look different— different in terms of weight goals, in terms of time taken, and in how they go about reaching them. That being said, there are some general guidelines given by the CDC (2022) as to how to go about achieving sustainable weight loss:

- **Make a commitment:** Write down these goals, and make sure they are visible daily.

- **Take stock of where you are:** Write down your current diet and when and why you waver from healthy eating (e.g., when moody, pressed for time, or around certain people).

- **Set realistic goals:** You might find it better to have both short-term goals (exercise for 100 minutes a week, replace soda with sugar-free iced tea, or cut down your portions of bread) and long-term goals (continue playing golf, continue to be able to go shopping by yourself, or even get fit enough to summit a specific mountain). Also, be realistic, specific (not just "lose weight" but rather "lose 10 lbs in one month"), and flexible (forgiving) in your goal settings.

- **Identify supporters:** Find like-minded people (e.g., family, friends, or groups) and resources (e.g., social media pages with encouraging messages, healthy recipes, or newsletters notifying you of nearby events you might enjoy) that will aid your journey to wellness.

- **Monitor progress:** Remember to take stock regularly. One day or a few days of failure doesn't spell defeat. Don't neglect to celebrate your successes and readjust goals as needed (e.g., increase your exercise minutes or cut down further on sugar if you started off only cutting down slightly).

Tend to focus on your long-term goals of eating healthy and exercising enough to continue doing what you enjoy, and weight management is kind of just a by-product of that lifestyle. I have found a simple analogy for this in the form of stock analysis.

Let's say you own a company. If you were to follow the movement of your company's stock price over five years, you may have observed its upward trend from $5 per share to $20 on a graphic representation for the five-year period. Most would consider this a success in the long term, right? Now consider if you were to zoom in on just the first year of activity. You may have seen fluctuations where the first six months may have read $5, $6, $7, $5, $6, and $6 despite you continuing to put resources into the company. Many people might stop here and consider the investment a failure, as the stock price only grew by $1. Over the next six months, the price might change again: $7, $9, $8, $11, $12, and closing on $12 for year one. By now, most would consider this a success as the investment more than doubled, correct?

If you zoom in deep enough, you'll find a two-week period where you gained 5 lbs. Yet, if you zoom out for that month, you remain constant. Always remember the bigger picture, and always keep your focus on the long-term goal. Continue to "put in the resources" (i.e., exercises and healthy eating), and in the bigger picture, probably without even realizing it, the weight will manage itself.

Now that you're aware of the *why* and the long-term outlook, I bet you're itching to know how you go about practically implementing chair exercises into your routine. Here are some tips that I myself and others have found helpful in starting new exercise routines:

- **Experiment:** Try out different exercise routines at different times of the day (morning vs. evening) for short periods of time (like one week) to see which works best.

- **Consistency**: If you're looking to have your healthy eating and exercise become a habit (without giving it much thought), you'll need to start by having it as a routine (scheduled frequently, intentionally, and repeatedly). The best way is to practice these things daily.

- **Start as simple as possible**: Every single person who has ever accomplished what you consider to be incredible had to start somewhere. The hardest part will be to show up on that chair—the rest will be history.

- **Get a workout buddy or group:** It is always a lot harder to cancel if you know your no-show is going to disappoint others.

- **Prepare:** Make things as easy as possible for yourself. Set out your workout clothing the night before, and set your chair in plain view so that there's no avoiding it. I, for example, often roll out my yoga mat next to my bed before I retire to bed. This way, there is no avoiding it the next morning.

- **Allow yourself flexibility:** No one is perfect. Simply do the best you can, and when you slip, get back into your routine as soon as possible. On days that you are struggling, try five minutes. Anything trumps nothing 100% of the time.

In closing, embarking on anything new in life is never easy. Additionally, the older you are, the harder this may be. But it is not impossible. The above will hopefully have provided you with enough tools to at least plan and start your journey. Knowing what has and has not worked for others is already as good a starting point as any. Throw in the fact that you should be able to tailor your goals as you need them, and you're all set to go.

Understanding Chair Exercises and the Benefits Of Them

The greatest miracle on earth is the human body.
It is stronger and wiser than you may realize,
and improving its ability to self-heal is within your control.
— Dr. Fabrizio Mancini

In this chapter, we will explore the benefits of chair exercises, as well as their impact on your body and why it's beneficial to practice them. By using these exercises regularly and sticking to a healthy eating plan, you will, without a doubt, soon start to see positive changes.

Neck rotation, extensions, and stretches help you improve posture, which worsens over the years, increase blood flow to the spinal cord, and relieve tension. Also, it boosts the strength of your neck. If you have a limited range of motion, it's important to remember not to force it. It's better to take it slowly and do it daily rather than once a week for an hour.

BENEFITS OF FRONT RAISES

Shoulder and chest muscles are strengthened through this isolation exercise, and definition on both the front and side of the shoulders will improve. This is vital for everyday life, as you use your shoulders to lift daily (e.g., lifting yourself out of a chair), and it has even been shown to reduce neck pain (Louw et al., 2017).

BENEFITS OF LATERAL RAISES

This specifically targets the deltoid's lateral and anterior heads. As with front raises, expect your shoulders to be strengthened and more flexible after doing these exercises regularly. With these raises, however, the left and right sides are worked independently, so discrepancies (between arms) can be corrected (Coratella et al., 2020). Doing these exercises regularly should also see your overall posture improve.

BENEFITS OF OVERHEAD PRESSES, BACK PRESSES, AND FRONT PRESSES

Overhead, back, and front presses are a great workout for your anterior deltoids, which are used whenever you perform an action that requires you to pull your shoulders back. An example would be when you need to reach for anything on a high shelf. Overhead presses are also probably one of the best exercises for improving your body's posture, even more so than lateral raises.

BENEFITS OF CORE STRENGTHENING EXERCISES

As explained earlier, the core muscles are made up of a group of muscles encompassing the entire torso. It consists of the abdomen muscles (front stomach), the obliques (internal and external side muscles), the transversus abdominis (the muscles surrounding the spine), the hips, and the lower back muscles. Some of the exercises that target the core include knee to elbow, extended leg raises, bicep curls, crossed arm crunches, and flutter kicks.

These exercises will play a pivotal role in improving the strength of your entire body; improving your balance, stability, and posture; assisting in making daily tasks like walking, getting out of bed, or standing up from a chair much easier; and assisting in reducing back and hip pain that plagues so many older adults.

BENEFITS OF SEATED CARDIO EXERCISES

Cardio exercises are an important part of any exercise routine as they get the heart pumping. By persistently doing these exercises, you will naturally decrease your resting heart rate and improve your heart muscles' ability to pump blood. In time, this will allow you to improve your exercise endurance. There are a host of other benefits for the body with all cardio exercises, which include lowering blood sugar, improving cholesterol, alleviating arthritic pains, and improving sleep and concentration.

Some examples of these exercises include seated jacks, lifts, leg lifts and twists, and chair running.

BENEFITS OF QUADRICEPS MUSCLE EXERCISES

Quadriceps refer to a group of four muscles (rectus femoris, vastus lateralis, vastus medialis, and vastus intermedius) running from the hips down to the front of the knee. The quadriceps are used in many of the daily activities we may take for granted. These include not only walking but also every time we either lower ourselves to sit or raise ourselves to stand up (e.g., using the bathroom). There are also benefits for the knees and hips, aiding posture, stability, and balance, as well as playing a role in decreasing the risk of osteoarthritis.

Some examples of these exercises include knee extensions, leg lifts, and sit-to-stand flow.

BENEFITS OF MODIFIED SUMO CHAIR AND CHAIR SQUATS

The sumo chair and chair squat modifications are, without a doubt, one of the best exercises for your leg muscles. They target muscles ranging from the lower back and gluteal muscles through the hamstrings and quadriceps. As mentioned above, these muscles are used for a variety of day-to-day activities, so it would be in your best interest not to neglect strengthening them.

How to Use This Book and Frequently Asked Questions

Take the first step in faith.
You don't have to see the whole staircase,
just take the first step.

— Martin Luther King, Jr.

In this book, you will find three different warm-up routines. To avoid routine fatigue, you can keep rotating them before you embark on the day's exercises. There are 28 different chair exercise routines and a cooldown stretch routine to complete after each session. As a bonus, if you scan the QR code at the start of the book, you will be able to access additional sequences for your wrists and ankles.

HOW TO USE THIS BOOK

1. Select one of the three warm-up options.
2. Select one of the 28 exercise sequences.
3. Do the cooldown stretches routine.

It's as simple as one, two, three. While not absolutely necessary, it is suggested you try all the different warm-ups on consecutive days (e.g., on day one, do warm-up one; on day two, do warm-up two; on day three, do warm-up three), and do the same with the workouts. Doing this will help you figure out not only which warm-ups and workouts are agreeable to your body but also which ones you enjoy more. You may, for example, find a certain sequence to be of great benefit to your lower back, so you might want to do that sequence at least twice a week.

The exercises do not require you to have any other equipment except for a chair. For a start, you will only be using your own body weight. For more advanced fitness levels, you can use weights for exercises that require them. Even this, though, does not require you to go out and buy dumbbells, as you can simply use filled water bottles or even soup cans.

For beginners, it is also essential that you listen to your body, not only while doing the exercises but also before and after. Observe the effects certain sequences have on your body, and if you start to find the exercises are becoming too easy, you can add weights to them (and don't hesitate to drop them when the exercises become too tough midway through either).

FREQUENTLY ASKED QUESTIONS

If I have health issues, can I still practice?

If you have any health concerns, it might be best to consult your doctor or a physician before you start. While most older adults should be able to complete these exercises without problems, there are certain situations where certain individuals might not be able to do them.

What kind of chair do I need?

You need a sturdy chair with no arms. The absence of arms allows for greater flexibility in movement, and the key is to select a chair that remains steadfast throughout your exercise routine, providing stability without shifting or moving. Choose any regular, sturdy chair for exercises; steer clear of folding chairs or those with wheels.

Do I need any other special gear or equipment?

You also don't need any special clothing or gear. Any clothing that allows you freedom of movement to complete the exercises should be fine. For more advanced exercises, you can consider using dumbbells, water bottles, or soup cans.

How often should I do the chair exercises?

Most adults should aim for at least 150 minutes of moderately intense exercise per week (CDC, 2019). This can be split up into two or three sessions per week or even daily. The guideline of 150 minutes can be increased slowly and safely, should your fitness levels allow.

How do I know if chair exercises are right for me?

Seated workouts are especially useful for the elderly, those who have trouble standing for longer periods of time and moving around, and, generally, those who suffer from balance issues. They can also be used as part of a complementary existing routine (e.g. if you're an active tennis player, golfer, or hiker). Still, the best way to know if something is right for you is to try it out!

Warm-ups and cooldowns

It is highly advisable to do both if you're to ensure injury is avoided. Warm-ups assist in warming your body temperature and muscles up slowly and safely. It is also considered a good way of signaling to your brain that the body is about to embark on physical activity—a sort of mental heads-up. Cooldown stretches also play a role in absorbing the benefits of the exercise you've done. It also helps in bringing your heart rate back down to its pre-workout state.

What is the core, and how do I engage it?

The core refers to a group of muscles centered around the abdomen, pelvis, spine, and diaphragm. It plays a pivotal role in just about every exercise you do. Without being physically present and showing you, it can be a bit tricky to explain. I've found the easiest way is the same way I was taught: While lying on your back on a flat surface (like the floor or bed), place your thumbs slightly below either side of your belly. Now, give a light cough. The area that experienced rapid expansion and contraction is where you want to focus on *engaging*. Keep your thumbs in place, and imagine a small ball is being placed in between your thumbs. To engage your core, the aim would be to move this imaginary ball from between your thumbs toward your chest without moving the rest of your body. Tilt only the belly area in the direction of your chest, and you should feel those muscles *engaged*.

ROOM

So now you are all set to start with the exercises. You'll want to ensure your workout area is clear of any sharp objects and other matter that could get in the way and interfere with your routine or even injure you. Lastly, make sure the exercise space is as tidy and calming as possible to avoid distractions. And with that, you can start planning for your first chair exercise session.

Initiating Your Chair Exercise Journey: Correct Posture

As you embark upon chair exercises for weight loss journey, it is important to observe your posture. Your body's positioning and alignment play an important role in the effectiveness of each exercise. At the same time, it ensures your comfort and safety throughout the process.

Sit comfortably with your spine straight. Visualize an imaginary line gently pulling you upwards from the top of your head, facilitating spinal elongation.

Elevate your head, ensuring your gaze is directed straight ahead. This helps maintain a healthy neck posture while simultaneously allowing chest expansion, crucial for improved respiration.

Always slightly tuck your chink in. When we age, we tend to stick our neck out.

Gently roll your shoulders back and allow them to relax. Activate your core muscles by drawing your belly button towards your spine. This will assist as a stabilizing center for all movements.

Bend your knees at a comfortable 90-degree angle with your feet flat on the floor. Allow your arms to rest gently on your lap.

Do this posture check before each session, starting with your warm-up routines.

Progressing Through Your Chair Exercise Journey

Now that you've mastered the art of perfect posture, you're all set to embark on the chair exercise routines designed for each day. It's essential to understand that these exercises are structured to cater to everyone, starting from a basic level. Whether you're a beginner or looking to challenge yourself further, there's a clear path for progression.

Starting With the Basics

You will find a different set of exercises for each day. These sets are basic to ensure you can perform them safely and effectively, focusing on technique and alignment.

How to Increase Difficulty

As you grow more comfortable and seek to intensify your workouts, here's how to progress:

Level One: This is your starting point. Simply follow the exercises as outlined for each day. Repeat them three times, allowing two minutes to rest between each set.

Level One Variation: To add a bit of a challenge, repeat each exercise for 30 seconds. You can either use your body weight or introduce weights into the routine. Suitable options include light dumbbells, soup cans, or water bottles, depending on your comfort and capability. Repeat them three times, allowing two minutes to rest between the exercise sets.

Level Two: Repeat the sequence five times for an increased challenge, allowing yourself two minutes of rest between exercise sets. It will boost the intensity and help to build endurance.

Level Three: To push your limits further, complete the sequence seven times with two minutes of rest between the sets. This level is designed to maximize your strength and endurance gains.

You can experiment by reducing rest time between sets, increasing exercise intensity, adding weights to the exercises, increasing the repetition of the exercises, or maybe you prefer to set the timer and repeat each exercise for 20 seconds, later rising to 30 seconds, and to 45 seconds or a minute! This is your oyster. Observe how you feel, familiarize yourself with the exercises, and create your routines. My created routines are a starting point for you.

Remember, the key to a successful fitness journey is progressing at a pace that feels right for you. Each level is designed to build upon the last, gradually increasing in intensity to foster improvement without risking injury. Listen to your body, and don't rush the process. Consistency and patience are your best allies as you advance through the levels.

By incorporating weights or increasing the duration and repetition of the exercises, you'll enhance the challenge and keep your workouts exciting and varied. Keep pushing your boundaries, and celebrate every step forward in this journey toward health and vitality.

THREE WARM-UP AND COOLDOWN ROUTINES

Warm-ups are an important part of the workout. It prepares the body to exercise. It increases blood flow, warms the muscles, and makes them more flexible. This is to reduce the risk of injuries. Warm-ups also gradually raise the heart rate, which helps with muscle efficiency and improves overall performance. They also help with mental reparation. Your brain and body know what is coming next. Warming up your body is essential to any exercise routine, contributing to safety and effectiveness.

Please type into your browser
https://www.youtube.com/@ZenflowHub

Then, select 'Playlists,' where you will see several playlists available. Choose the one relevant to your book title, such as *28 Days of Chair Yoga for Seniors for Weight Loss*.

Or scan QR Code which will take you directly to the playlist

These videos are designed to assist you in performing the exercises detailed in this book. They serve as a valuable resource for checking your form or for additional clarification on the exercise techniques. The demonstrations include all exercises covered in the book, from warm-ups to main workout routines.

WARM-UP ONE

Before starting your warm-up routine, check your body's alignment first.

Sit and look up straight. Keep your chin ever so slightly tucked in.

Roll your shoulders back. Keep them relaxed. Lengthen your neck. Engage your core's stability. This is important for the exercise routines. Knees are bent at 90 degrees, and arms rest on your laps.

Neck Stretch

Keep your chin slightly tucked in. Turn your head gently to the right and then gently to the left. Hold the stretch for two to three seconds before moving your head to the opposite side. Repeat the same, moving your head up and down. Repeat three times in each direction—left, right, up, and down.

Shoulder Circles

Bring fingertips to shoulders—circle six to eight times in each direction. If you have limited mobility in your shoulders, then do only half of the circle.

Shoulder Stretch

Bring your hands behind the head. Pull your elbows back as much as possible; imagine your shoulder blades having to keep a pencil between them. And then slowly move your elbows forward, trying to touch each other. Repeat the movement three to five times.

Lateral Arm Raises

Raise your arms parallel to the ground and at shoulder height, and lower them back to your sides. Feel your abdominal wall engaged, and don't hinge in the shoulders. Repeat the movement eight to ten times.

Upper Body Twist

Engage your core. Keep the chin slightly tucked in. Cross your

arms on your chest and twist to the right. Return to the center, and then twist to the left. Alternate and repeat five to eight times.

Knee Extension

Extend your leg parallel to the floor or at the height that is comfortable for you. Feel your quadriceps muscles working on the front of the thigh. Repeat five to eight times, and then switch sides.

Ankle Circles

Lift your foot up a few inches from the floor, keeping your knee straight. Rotate the ankle one side three to five times, then in the opposite direction. Repeat the exercise with another leg.

Marching on the Spot

March on the spot, counting a total of 30 steps.

Now, you should be all warmed up and can continue your daily exercise routine. (Day 1, Day 2, etc.)

WARM-UP TWO

Neck Stretch

Keep your chin slightly tucked in. Turn your head gently to the right and then gently to the left. Hold the stretch for two to three seconds before moving your head to the opposite side. Repeat the same, moving your head up and down. Repeat three times in each direction—left, right, up, and down.

Shoulder Rolls

Keep the arms on your lap or next to you. Lift your shoulders and roll them back three times, then move them in the opposite direction.

Chest Stretch

Begin by sitting tall, away from the back of the chair. Roll your shoulders back and down. Extend your arms to the sides, then gently press your chest forward and upward, savoring the stretch across your chest. Hold this position for five to eight seconds, and repeat it three to five times.

Upper Body Twist

Engage your core. Keep the chin slightly tucked in. Cross your arms on your chest and twist to the right. Return to the center, and then twist to the left. Alternate and repeat six to eight times.

Flexing Foot

Lift your leg. Point the toes away from you. Pull the toes toward your chest and press the heel away. Repeat five to eight times before switching to the other leg.

Marching on the Spot

March on the spot, counting a total of 30 steps.

WARM-UP THREE

Neck Rolls

Start with small circles and roll your neck to the right side, slowly increasing the circle. The reverse—start with a big circle and get down to a small one, where you started. Repeat it once or twice.

Shoulder Shrugs

Inhale and raise your shoulders toward your earlobes. Keep your hands perpendicular to the floor throughout the exercise. Repeat six to eight times.

Arm Circles

Extend your arms to your sides. Keep them parallel to the floor at shoulder height. Slowly start to make small circles and keep increasing them. Complete five to eight moves in one direction and, when reversed, start with big circles and reduce them back to small circles.

Heel Raises

With your feet flat on the ground, lift your heels as high as you can off of the ground. You can do both legs or alternate. Repeat ten to fifteen times for each leg.

Front Punches

Keep your abdominals engaged. Bend your arms up so your wrists are by your shoulders. With control, slowly punch in front of, up, and across your body with one arm while slightly rotating your torso in the same direction. Return to the start position, then switch to the other arm. Alternate and repeat twenty times.

Overhead Punches

Bend your arms, and with control, slowly punch above your head with one arm. Fully straighten it, or as much as you can, and bring it down. Switch to the other arm. Alternate and repeat twenty times.

Run on the Spot

Instead of marching, run as fast as you can on the spot for 30 seconds.

Now, you should be all warmed up and can continue your daily exercise routine. (Day 1, Day 2, etc.)

COOLDOWN ROUTINE

Cooldowns are a no less important part of the workout routine than warm-ups. Adding the cooldown routine to your workout helps your body slowly return to normal. Slowing down the heart rate and breathing reduces the risk of dizziness or fainting after intense exercise. Cooldowns are essential for easing muscle stiffness and soreness by helping to eliminate lactic acid buildup. They allow for muscle stretching, which enhances flexibility and prevents injuries. Cooldowns also give a moment for mental relaxation, signaling to your brain and body that the workout is complete.

Cross Body Shoulder Stretch

Take one arm and place it across your chest. Using your other hand, take the outer forearm of the arm that's across your body. Push that arm into your body to feel more of a stretch. Remain in the position for thirty seconds. Repeat with the other arm.

Triceps Stretch

When sitting down or standing up, roll your shoulders back.

Reach your right arm upward, then flex at the elbow to guide the right palm toward the middle of your back, placing your middle finger along your spine. Let your left hand guide your elbow toward the center and downward. Stay in this stretch for thirty seconds. Repeat it four times on each side.

Upward Hand Stretch

Bring your arms in front and lengthen. Interlock your fingers with palms facing outside and raise your arms above your head. Keep fingers softly locked. Remain in the stretch for about three to four breaths. Repeat twice.

Forward Fold

On the inhale, raise your arms up and gently stretch. On the exhale, take the arms toward your feet, with the torso resting on the thighs and chin close to the knees. Feel a stretch across your shoulders and back. To release, inhale, look up first, then raise your arms before returning to sit. Remain in the pose for two breaths or till you feel comfortable.

Note: If you have high blood pressure or difficulty breathing, you should not do this pose.

Hamstring Stretch

Sit closer to the front of the chair. Extend one leg in front of you, pulling the toes toward you. Lean as far as you can. Feel the hamstring stretch. Remain for two to three breaths. Switch the legs

Leg Stretch

Sit on the chair and extend your legs with your heels on the ground. Place your hands behind your head, keep your elbows out and shoulders rolled back. Look forward.

Hinge from your waist; keep your back straight, and lower your upper body as far as possible. Feel the stretch behind your legs.

Keep here for three to five breaths and return to a sitting position.

Seated Quad Stretch

Move to the left side of your chair. Keep the right leg on the chair and bring the left foot back. Feel the stretch in your left quad. If you don't feel it, then gently lean back into it. Stay in the position for a few breaths and repeat on the opposite side.

Seated Figure Four or Pigeon Pose

Put your right ankle over the left knee or on the left shin. With your back straight, lean forward and remain for a few breaths, feeling the stretch in your hip. Repeat on the other side.

DAY 1

Seated Arm Flow

Bring both arms in front of you with palms touching. Leave left arm in front of you as the right opens parallel to the shoulder-level floor. Move your head to the right. Return the right arm to the middle and repeat to the opposite side—alternate and repeat ten to twelve times.

Arm Swings

Allow your arms to swing forward, hands crossing over each other. Swing arms back, then forward again, alternating which hand swings over the top of the other. Continue the movement ten to twelve times.

Front Arm Raise

Lift your arms above your head in coordination with lifting your heels. Lower the arms halfway in front of you, at shoulder level, with palms facing each other. Lower the heels simultaneously with the arms. Repeat eight to ten times.

Leg and Arm Lift

Engage your core with the belly button pulled in. Raise both arms and lift one leg and lower. Alternate and repeat twelve to fourteen times.

Torso Twist with Straight Arms

Straighten your arms in front of you, join the palms together—alternate twisting to the sides. Repeat ten to twelve times.

Seated Shoulder Press

You can use weights if you want to, as this depends on your physical abilities. Using your body weight is also great for the workout. Engage the core muscles.

Begin with both elbows extended to the sides under the shoulders, chest lifted. Face forward with palms turned outward. Extend the arms upward, reaching above the head until fully extended or to a comfortable range. Avoid touching the hands together, and keep both arms parallel. Gradually lower the hands to the starting position and maintain spread elbows. Avoid tucking the elbows toward the body's center; extend them outward until a gentle pinching sensation (not painful) is felt at the shoulder blades' top. Repeat eight to ten times.

Modified Jumping Jacks

Move closer to the front of the chair with arms at your sides. In a harmonious motion, lift your arms overhead, fingertips gently meeting, with palms turned outward. Simultaneously, extend one leg outward with toes touching the ground as your arms ascend. Bring the extended leg back to the center as you lower your arms. Alternate and repeat eighteen to twenty times.

Skip Rope

Rope skipping—imitate rope skipping using an imaginary rope.

Repeat thirty times.

Your first day is completed.
I hope you enjoyed it. Don't forget to do your cooldown routine.

DAY 2

Seated Shoulder Press

You can use weights if you want to, as this depends on your physical abilities. Using your body weight is also great for the workout. Engage the core muscles.

Begin with both elbows extended to the sides under the shoulders, chest lifted. Face forward with palms turned outward. Extend the arms upward, reaching above the head until fully extended or to a comfortable range. Avoid touching the hands together, and keep both arms parallel. Gradually lower the hands to the starting position and maintain spread elbows. Avoid tucking the elbows toward the body's center; extend them outward until a gentle pinching sensation (not painful) is felt at the shoulder blades' top. Repeat eight to ten times.

Lateral Arm Raises

Ensure your back is straight. Engage your abs. Place your arms down by your sides. Slowly lift them with weight or without parallel to the ground at shoulder level. Slowly lower them down. Repeat eight to ten times.

Seated Knee Extension

Extend your leg parallel to the floor or at the height that is comfortable for you. Feel your quadriceps muscles working on the front of the thigh. Repeat one leg six to eight times, and then switch the sides.

Do two sets for each leg.

Elbow to Knee

Keep feet flat on the floor and shoulders rolled back. Feel your abs engaged. Place your hands behind your head, elbows pointing out to the sides. Lift your right knee toward your chest while simultaneously bringing the left elbow toward your right knee. Return to the starting position with control. Repeat on the opposite side. Alternate and repeat eight to ten times.

Kick and Clap

Extend one leg forward with a controlled kick, clapping your hands at shoulder height. Focus on utilizing your thigh muscles and ensuring a smooth, deliberate motion. Engage your core and kick with force, maintaining a consistent pace. Alternate legs and repeat the sequence twenty to twenty-four times.

Tap and Reach

Extend one arm diagonally as you stretch the leg on the same side in the opposite direction. Reach your fingertips toward the ceiling, lengthening the arm while stretching the leg. Focus on executing smooth, controlled movements, aiming to create a straight line from your fingertips to your toes. Alternate legs and repeat the sequence twenty to twenty-four times.

Seated Jacks

Move closer to the front of the chair with arms at your sides. In a harmonious motion, lift your arms overhead, fingertips gently meeting, with palms turned outward. Simultaneously, extend both legs out as your arms ascend. Bring both legs back to the center as your arms land. Repeat eight to ten times.

If extending both legs and arms simultaneously is too challenging, try this version instead.

Observe your breathing and body. Do it at a pace that suits you.

Try not to hold your breath.

DAY 3

Front Punches

Maintain an upright posture. Engage your core, chest, and arm muscles, ensuring a firm contraction with each swing. Position your lightly clenched fists close to your jawline. With control, slowly punch in front and return to the start position, then switch to the other arm. Alternate and repeat twenty times.

Punch Down

Maintain an upright posture. Engage your core, chest, and arm muscles, ensuring a firm contraction with each swing. Bend your arms and make a fist. With control, slowly punch down and return to the start position, then switch to the other arm. Alternate and repeat twenty times.

Front Punches

Maintain an upright posture. Engage your core, chest, and arm muscles, ensuring a firm contraction with each swing. Position your lightly clenched fists close to your jawline. With control, slowly punch in front and return to the start position, then switch to the other arm. Alternate and repeat twenty times.

Upper Cuts

Sit up with your back straight and keep your feet flat on the floor. Place your hands close to your sides, forming two clenched fists facing you. Bend your elbows, pulling your fists in closer to your body. Punch each fist in an upward motion. Aim to stop the punch around chin level. Minimize unnecessary movement in the upper body. Encourage controlled breathing, exhaling with each punch. As mentioned above, controlled motion to avoid punching yourself in the face. (Real story and experience.)

Alternate between your right and left hand for each punch—repeat twenty times.

Start with a slow and controlled pace, then gradually increase speed as comfortable.

Overhead Punches

With control, slowly punch above your head with one arm. Return to the start position, then switch to the other arm. Alternate and repeat twenty times on each side.

DAY 4

Lateral Arm Raises

Ensure your back is straight. Engage your abs. Place your arms down by your sides. Slowly lift them with weight or without parallel to the ground at shoulder level. Slowly lower them down. Repeat eight to ten times.

Hinge and Cross

Sit straight with knees bent and heels lifted. Squeeze the inner thighs together for more muscular activation. Place hands behind the head and engage your core. Lean back until the shoulder blades lightly touch the back of the chair.

Bring your body forward, crossing your right elbow to the outside of your left knee. Return to start. Repeat for twenty alternating reps.

Extended Leg Raises

Engage your abs and lean back about 45 degrees. Feel your abs tighten.

Grab the sides of the chair if you need to. Stretch both legs in front of you and lift one leg. Feel your lower abdominals working. Lower it down and then lift the opposite leg. Alternate and repeat sixteen to twenty times.

Seated Side Step Over

Lift your right knee and step over the imaginary object on the floor. Lift the leg and step over it. Bring it back by stepping over back. Repeat for eight to twelve repetitions before switching to the opposite leg.

Tap and Reach

Extend one arm diagonally as you stretch the leg on the same side in the opposite direction. Reach your fingertips toward the ceiling, lengthening the arm while stretching the leg. Focus on executing smooth, controlled movements, aiming to create a straight line from your fingertips to your toes. Alternate legs and repeat the sequence twenty to twenty-four times.

Chair Squat

Start with your knees shoulder-width apart. Lean forward and lift your hips off the chair. If needed, you can hold the chair's edges for support as you safely return to the seated position. Alternatively, place your arms on your knees, but avoid leaning into them. Engage your glutes and hamstrings to assist in lifting your hips. Repeat this movement ten times.

DAY 5

Kick and Toe Touch

Take a short break if you need to. Keep the arms behind your head. Ensure you're not putting all the arm's weight and forcing your neck down. Keep your back straight and core engaged. Arms behind the head. Lift the leg and extend the opposite arm, trying to reach the toes of the opposite leg while the other arm stays behind the head. Alternate and repeat twelve to fourteen times.

Bicycle Curls

Lean back into the chair and grab the edges of the chair. Extend one leg out and pull the knee back to your chest. Think if you're peddling the bicycle. Repeat on one side six to eight times. Switch to the opposite side. Now reverse—start with one leg peddling in the opposite direction. Switch sides and repeat six to eight times.

Single March with a Twist

Lean back into the chair with your back straight; don't round your back. Move the bottom toward the edge of the chair. You can hold the edges of the chair with your arms. Core engaged. Do single marches by lifting your knee as high as you can. Alternate and repeat ten to fourteen times.

If you're feeling brave and strong, lift both knees simultaneously. Repeat six to eight times.

Flutter Kicks

Lean back into the chair with your spine straight. Fully extend your legs, hold the chair's edges, lift both legs, and flutter. Kick your legs up and down. Repeat twenty times.

Chair Pose Above Chair

Maintain an upright posture and lift your arms above your head while exhaling deeply. Inhale and move into a chair pose, gently raising yourself to your feet above the chair. Exhale and return to a seated position, arms still extended overhead. Inhale again and resume the chair pose. Repeat this sequence six times to ten times.

DAY 6

Modify Chair Squat

Start with your knees shoulder-width apart. Lean forward and lift your hips off the chair. If needed, you can hold the chair's edges for support as you safely return to the seated position.

Alternatively, place your arms on your knees, but avoid leaning into them. Engage your glutes and hamstrings to assist in lifting your hips. Repeat this movement ten times.

Straight Leg Raise Twist

Position yourself at the front of the chair. Extend your right leg while ensuring your left foot stays grounded. Cross your arms over your chest and engage your abdominal muscles..Rotate your torso to the right, lifting your right leg.

Squeeze your knees together and return to the starting position.

Switch sides and repeat. Alternate and repeat sixteen to twenty repetitions.

Seated Jacks with Straight Arms

Put the palms together with straight arms in front of you. Hold your knees together. Move closer to the front of the chair if you need to.

Open your arms to the sides and step the right foot out to the sides. Open your hips as much as you can. Arms are returning to the middle, the same as the right foot. Alternate and repeat a total of twenty times.

Lateral and Front Arm Raises

Ensure your back is straight. Engage your abs. Place your arms down by your sides. Slowly lift them with weight or without parallel to the ground at shoulder level. Slowly lower them down. Lift them in front of you—shoulder level and lower them down. Control the movement; don't swing your arms. Repeat eight to ten times. You can add weights.

Seat Hollow body

Come to the front of the chair, and with your back straight, raise your arms. Lean back at about a 45-degree angle. You should feel a contraction in your abdominals. If it feels too much with your hands over your head, cross the arms on your chest and hold. Focus on your abs. Maintain the back straight and keep leaning back.

Slowly count to 30. Take a few breaths, rest, and repeat it.

Elbow to Knee

Keep feet flat on the floor and shoulders rolled back. Feel your abs engaged. Place your hands behind your head, elbows pointing out to the sides. Lift your right knee toward your chest while simultaneously bringing the left elbow toward your right knee. Return to the starting position with control. Repeat on the opposite side. Alternate and repeat eight to ten times.

DAY 7

Chair Mountain Climbers Variation

Lean back at a 45-degree angle. Brace yourself on the chair and bring your bottom right to the very front of it. Extend your legs out and get one knee to the chest as best as you possibly can. Maintain a 45-degree position with your upper body. Don't turn this into a crunch. Keep your torso straight, and only your knees are coming toward your chest. Alternate and repeat twenty times.

Side Raise and Knee Raise

Keep both legs on the floor with knees bent at a 90-degree angle. Bend your elbows and lift them parallel to the floor at shoulder height. Simultaneously, lift one knee up. Bring the elbows and the knee back down. Repeat with the opposite knee—lift the elbows up with the opposite knee. Alternate and repeat twenty times. You can use weights for this movement.

Upper-Body Twist

Engage your core. Keep the chin slightly tucked in. Cross your arms on your chest and twist to the right. Return to the center and then twist to the left. Alternate and repeat eight to ten times.

Sumo Chair Get Up

The feet are wider than the hips, and the toes point out slightly. Place your arms in front of you on the chair, lean slightly forward, and lift yourself, but don't fully stand up. Feel your feet firmly on the floor. Don't place the weight onto your hands—the thigh muscles are holding the weight. If you want to make it harder, remove the hands from the chair. Thighs are parallel to the floor. Repeat ten times.

Triceps Extensions

Lean forward at 45 degrees with the spine straight. Bend the elbows and pull them slightly back. Extend your arm back from your elbow; think you are flexing at the elbow joint. If you're working out with weights (bottles or soup cans) that feel too much, drop them and carry on with the movement with no weights. Repeat fourteen to sixteen times.

Seat Hollow Body

Come to the front of the chair, and with your back straight, raise your arms. Lean back at about a 45-degree angle. You should feel a contraction in your abdominals. If it feels too much with your hands over your head, cross the arms on your chest and hold. Focus on your abs. Maintain the back straight and keep leaning back.

Slowly count to 30. Take a few breaths, rest, and repeat it.

DAY 8

Front Kick and Punch

Maintain an upright posture. Engage your core. Keep your feet shoulder-width apart. Position your lightly clenched fists close to your jawline. With control, slowly punch in front of, up, and across your body with one arm while slightly rotating your torso in the same direction. Simultaneously, kick the opposite leg out. Alternate and repeat twenty times. You can use weights to increase the punch intensity if you need to.

Chair Squat

Start with your knees shoulder-width apart. Lean forward and lift your hips off the chair. If needed, you can hold the chair's edges for support as you safely return to the seated position. Alternatively, place your arms on your knees, but avoid leaning into them. Engage your glutes and hamstrings to assist in lifting your hips. Repeat this movement ten times.

Leg and Arm Lift

Bend your arms and keep them close to your body. It's similar to a marching move. Instead of alternating, you work the same leg. The arm goes up, and the opposite knee goes toward your chest. Lift your left knee with the right arm. Repeat ten times for each leg.

Straight Leg Raise Twist

Position yourself at the front of the chair.

Extend your right leg while ensuring your left foot stays grounded.

Cross your arms over your chest and engage your abdominal muscles.

Rotate your torso to the right, lifting your right leg.

Squeeze your knees together and return to the starting position. Switch sides and repeat. Alternate and repeat sixteen to twenty repetitions.

Hot Feet and Bicep Curl

Sit with your knees slightly apart and elbows next to your body. Start quickly running on the spot—as if the ground would feel hot, lightly tap your soles, and then incorporate a bicep curl.

Keep elbows bent at your side, turn your palms up, extend both your arms, and curl. Repeat eight to ten times.

DAY 9

Leg and Arm Lift

Bend your arms and keep them close to your body. It's similar to a marching move. Instead of alternating, you work the same leg. The arm goes up, and the opposite knee goes toward your chest. Lift your left knee with the right arm. Repeat ten times for each leg.

Leg Extension and Arm Crossover

Legs are shoulder-width apart. Arms are straight crossed in front of you, perpendicular to the floor. Extend the heel out simultaneously as you uncross the arms and take them to your sides, parallel to the ground. Take the heel back in and cross your arms. Repeat—uncross the arms, kick the heel out, and bring them back. Alternate the legs and repeat twenty times.

Seesaw Row

Keep your legs hip-width apart. Lean slightly forward with a straight back. The arms are straight and in between your legs. Bend the elbow and pull it back. Lower the arms back. Alternate and repeat twenty times. When you are ready, use weights.

Dumbbell Curl and Kick

Feet hip apart. Kick the right leg out and bring it back. Kick the left leg out and get it back. Hold your arm with a dumbbell with your palm facing upward. If you're not using a weight, imagine that you're holding it up. Slowly curl the weight up (or just your arm) by bending your elbow, keeping your elbow close to your body. Then, slowly lower the weight to the starting position. Now add the kick—curl both arms and right-left kick and keep alternating legs and coordinating with a bicep curl movement. Repeat twenty times.

High and Low Pulls

Keep knees hip-width apart. Sit with your back straight. Imagine the rope above your head—extend the right arm up and pull it down. Keep your elbows next to the ribcage. Then, fully extend your left arm and repeat the same move. Both elbows at your ribcage.

Lean slightly forward and repeat the following movement below your knees as if you are pulling something up from the ground. Utilize both your right and left arms to execute the pulling motion. The sequence consists of four moves: first, pull down with your left and right arms, then pull up with your right arm, followed by your left arm. Repeat this sequence fourteen to eighteen times.

DAY 10

Push and Step to the Side

Sit in the middle of the chair, closer to the edge of the seat.

Step the right leg out and, simultaneously, push both arms out in front of you, stretch out, the palms and fingers facing up. Pull your arms back to your sides when the leg returns to the center.

Emphasize the push-out and pull-back arm movement—thirty movements in total.

Torso Twist

Put your arms behind your head and keep your elbows wide. Feel your abdominals engaged, gently twist, return to the center, and turn on another side. Alternate and repeat ten to fourteen times.

Running on the Spot

Instead of marching, run as fast as you can on the spot for 30 seconds.

Dumbbell Curl and Kick

Feet hip apart. Kick the right leg out and bring it back. Kick the left leg out and get it back. Hold your arm with a dumbbell with your palm facing upward. If you're not using a weight, imagine that you're holding it up. Slowly curl the weight up (or just your arm) by bending your elbow, keeping your elbow close to your body. Then, slowly lower the weight to the starting position. Now add the kick—curl both arms and right-left kick and keep alternating legs and coordinating with a bicep curl movement. Repeat twenty times.

Front Punches

Keep your abdominals engaged. Bend your arms up so your wrists are by your shoulders. With control, slowly punch in front of, up, and across your body with one arm while slightly rotating your torso in the same direction. Return to the start position, then switch to the other arm. Alternate and repeat twenty times.

Split Squat Variation

Move closer toward the front of the chair.

Lean back about 45 degrees. If you need to, then hold the edges of the chair. Bring your knee to your chest as close as possible, push it out by straightening it, and bring it back to your chest. Keep repeating this movement for eight to twelve times. Switch the legs, repeat.

Mindfully extend your leg rather than kicking it out. Push it out and bring it in.

Back Bend

Sit nice and tall at the chair's edge with your knees bent. Elbows are bent at 90-degree angles next to your ribcage. Now lean forward from your hips with a straight back, ensuring the head is aligned with your back. Return to the sitting position. Repeat this movement ten to fifteen times. You can hold weights if you can.

DAY 11

Marching and Arm Circles

Start marching on the spot. Extend your arms to your sides. Keep them parallel to the floor at shoulder height. Slowly start to make small circles and keep increasing them. Complete five to eight moves in one direction and, when reversed, start with big circles, and reduce them back to small circles.

Side Reach

Keep your knees at the shoulder width.

Reach with the right arm up and lean slightly to the left side. Feel the side stretch. Keep alternating and repeat twenty times in total.

Front Reach

Now energetically, keep reaching to the front, slightly angling at the opposite side. Keep alternating and counting a total of twenty moves.

Elbow to Knee

Keep feet flat on the floor and shoulders rolled back. Feel your abs engaged. Place your hands behind your head, elbows pointing out to the sides. Lift your right knee toward your chest while simultaneously bringing the left elbow toward your right knee. Return to the starting position with control. Repeat on the opposite side. Alternate and repeat eight to ten times.

Skater Switch

Shift to the front of your chair.

Bend your right knee while extending your left leg to the opposite side.

Keep your toes pointed.

Start extending your arms. Lean forward and attempt to reach the inside of your right foot with your left arm. Swiftly switch and repeat the movement with the right arm and the left foot. The back is straight. Alternate sides and repeat twenty-five to thirty times.

Straight Leg Raise Twist

Position yourself at the front of the chair.

Extend your right leg while ensuring your left foot stays grounded.

Cross your arms over your chest and engage your abdominal muscles.

Rotate your torso to the right, lifting your right leg.

Squeeze your knees together and return to the starting position.

Switch sides and repeat. Alternate and repeat sixteen to twenty repetitions.

DAY 12

Stand Up Flow

Keep your feet flat on the floor, shoulder-width apart, and underneath your hips. Keep your back and neck straight, with your chest slightly forward. Lean forward and slightly shift your weight to the front of your feet. Slowly stand up. Try not to support any weight with your hands. Take a full breath, and tighten your core and abdominal muscles to control your lowering as much as possible. Lower yourself to the chair with control. Repeat six to ten times.

Heel Raises

Sit with your back straight. Ensure that both your feet are straight and the toes are facing forward. The alignment is important.

Lift your heel. Repeat each leg ten times before switching to the opposite side.

Skip Rope

Rope skipping—imitate rope skipping using an imaginary rope.

Repeat thirty times.

Plank Pose with Chair

Place your hands on the seat of the chair. Stack shoulders over hands, walk your feet back, hip-distance apart. Depending on your body's abilities, walk your feet as far as you feel comfortable. You can be on your toes or feet flat, core engaged. Observe your shoulders being stacked over your wrists. Keep your spine straight. Long line from shoulders to feet. Hold five long, deep breaths or less.

Seated Knee Swirls

Keep your knees together.

Sit in an upright position with your knees together and hold the edges of the chair. Swivel your knees to the side. Keep doing this for eight to ten times.

Side-to-Side Punches

Keep knees hip-width apart.

Maintain an upright posture. Engage your core, chest, and arm muscles, ensuring a firm contraction with each swing. Position your lightly clenched fists. With control, slowly punch in front of, up, and across your body with one arm while slightly rotating your torso in the same direction. Return to the start position, then switch to the other arm. Alternate and repeat twenty times.

DAY 13

Torso Twist

ut your arms behind your head and keep your elbows wide. Feel your abdominals engaged, gently twist, return to the center, and turn on another side. Alternate and repeat ten to fourteen times.

Elbow to Knee

Keep feet flat on the floor and shoulders rolled back. Feel your abs engaged. Place your hands behind your head, elbows pointing out to the sides. Lift your right knee toward your chest while simultaneously bringing the left elbow toward your right knee. Return to the starting position with control. Repeat on the opposite side. Alternate and repeat eight to ten times.

Bicycle Curls

Lean back into the chair and grab the edges of the chair. Extend one leg out and pull the knee back to your chest. Think if you're peddling the bicycle. Repeat on one side six to eight times. Switch to the opposite side. Now reverse—start with one leg peddling in the opposite direction. Switch sides and repeat six to eight times.

Crossed Arms Crunches

Sit with your back straight and core engaged. Cross the arms on your chest. Now lean back, feel your abs working, and using the abbs, bring yourself back to the straight sit-up position. Repeat eight to ten times.

Side Reaches

Sit up straight. Reach the right arm up and reach it over. Feel the stretch and pull yourself back up. Alternate and repeat eight to ten times.

Single March with a Twist

Lean back into the chair with your back straight; don't round your back. Move the bottom toward the edge of the chair. You can hold the edges of the chair with your arms. Core engaged. Do single marches by lifting your knee as high as you can. Alternate and repeat ten to fourteen times.

If you're feeling brave and strong, lift both knees simultaneously. Repeat six to eight times.

DAY 14

Marching on the Spot

March on the spot, counting a total of 50 steps.

Seated Shoulder Press

You can use weights if you want to, as this depends on your physical abilities. Using your body weight is also great for the workout. Engage the core muscles.

Begin with both elbows extended to the sides under the shoulders, chest lifted. Face forward with palms turned outward. Extend the arms upward, reaching above the head until fully extended or to a comfortable range. Avoid touching the hands together and keep both arms parallel. Gradually lower the hands to the starting position and maintain spread elbows. Avoid tucking the elbows toward the body's center; extend them outward until a gentle pinching sensation (not painful) is felt at the shoulder blades' top. Repeat eight to ten times.

Star Crunch

Sitting on the edge of the seat, bring your arms above your head. Stretch your legs out with heels digging into the ground. Bring your right elbow to meet your left knee and return to the start position. Repeat on the opposite side. Keep your spine straight and repeat alternating fourteen to sixteen times.

Extended Leg Circles

Sit up straight and lean back into the back of the chair. Kick the leg out (lifted). Pull your leg toward your chest and lean forward to meet your knee. Repeat five to eight times for each leg.

Side-to-Side Punches

Maintain an upright posture. Engage your core, chest, and arm muscles, ensuring a firm contraction with each swing. Position your lightly clenched fists. With control, slowly punch in front of, up, and across your body with one arm while slightly rotating your torso in the same direction. Return to the start position, then switch to the other arm. Alternate and repeat twenty times.

Overhead Punches

Bend your arms, and with control, slowly punch above your head with one arm. Fully straighten it, or as much as you can, and bring it down. Switch to the other arm. Alternate and repeat twenty times.

Leg Extensions with a Twist

Lean slightly back and hold the edges of the chair. This is a four-step exercise:

Lift your knee toward your chest, and kick the leg by straightening it out. Then, please bring it back to your chest and lower it on the floor. Work on one leg before switching to the opposite side. Repeat six to eight times.

Sumo Chair Get Up

The feet are wider than the hips, and the toes point out slightly. Place your arms in front of you on the chair, lean slightly forward, and lift yourself, but don't fully stand up. Feel your feet firmly on the floor. Don't place the weight onto your hands—the thigh muscles are holding the weight. If you want to make it harder, remove the hands from the chair. Thighs are parallel to the floor. Repeat ten times.

DAY 15

High and Low Pulls

Keep knees hip-width apart. Sit with your back straight. Imagine the rope above your head—extend the right arm up and pull it down. Keep your elbows next to the ribcage. Then, fully extend your left arm and repeat the same move. Both elbows at your ribcage.

Lean slightly forward and repeat the following movement below your knees as if you are pulling something up from the ground. Utilize both your right and left arms to execute the pulling motion. The sequence consists of four moves: first, pull down with your left and right arms, then pull up with your right arm, followed by your left arm. Repeat this sequence fourteen to eighteen times.

Lateral and Front Arm Raises

Ensure your back is straight. Engage your abs. Place your arms down by your sides. Slowly lift them with weight or without parallel to the ground at shoulder level. Slowly lower them down. Lift them in front of you—shoulder level and lower them down. Control the movement; don't swing your arms. Repeat eight to ten times. You can add weights.

Tap and Reach

Extend one arm diagonally as you stretch the leg on the same side in the opposite direction. Reach your fingertips toward the ceiling, lengthening the arm while stretching the leg. Focus on executing smooth, controlled movements, aiming to create a straight line from your fingertips to your toes. Alternate legs and repeat the sequence twenty to twenty-four times.

Modify Chair Squat

Start with your knees shoulder-width apart. Lean forward and lift your hips off the chair. If needed, you can hold the chair's edges for support as you safely return to the seated position. Alternatively, place your

arms on your knees, but avoid leaning into them. Engage your glutes and hamstrings to assist in lifting your hips. Repeat this movement ten times.

Kick and Toe Touch

Take a short break if you need to. Keep the arms behind your head. Ensure you're not putting all the arm's weight and forcing your neck down. Keep your back straight and core engaged. Arms behind the head. Lift the leg and extend the opposite arm, trying to reach the toes of the opposite leg while the other arm stays behind the head. Alternate and repeat twelve to fourteen times.

DAY 16

Marching on the Spot

March on the spot, counting a total of 50 steps.

Lateral Arm Raises

Ensure your back is straight. Engage your abs. Place your arms down by your sides. Slowly lift them with weight or without parallel to the ground at shoulder level. Slowly lower them down. Repeat eight to ten times.

Knee Extension

Extend your leg parallel to the floor or at the height that is comfortable for you. Feel your quadriceps muscles working on the front of the thigh. Repeat eight to ten times and then switch the sides.

Back Rows

Sit up straight. Bend forward at 45 degrees. Keep your arms straight next to your sides with knuckles facing outward. Raise your arms by sticking your elbows out. Repeat eight to ten times.

Hip Openers

Sit up straight. Engage your core. Keep your knees together, your arms on your thighs. Open the knees to the sides and return them to the starting point. Repeat sixteen to twenty times.

Upright Row

Hold your arms with palms facing toward you at your side. Initiate a gradual lift of the arms, letting elbows lead the movement. Elbows are moving up. Try not to lift the shoulders—only the elbows. Slowly lower it down. Lift your elbows. It's a controlled lift. Lower it down. Repeat eight to twelve times.

Sumo Chair Get Up

The feet are wider than the hips, and the toes point out slightly. Place your arms in front of you on the chair, lean slightly forward, and lift yourself, but don't fully stand up. Feel your feet firmly on the floor. Don't place the weight onto your hands—the thigh muscles are holding the weight. If you want to make it harder, remove the hands from the chair. Thighs are parallel to the floor. Repeat ten times.

Chair Mountain Climbers Variation

Lean back at a 45-degree angle. Brace yourself on the chair and bring your bottom right to the very front of it. Extend your legs out and get one knee to the chest as best as you possibly can. Maintain a 45-degree position with your upper body. Don't turn this into a crunch. Keep your torso straight, and only your knees are coming toward your chest. Alternate and repeat twenty times.

Your sixteenth day is completed. Don't forget to do your cooldown routine.

DAY 17

Front Punches

Maintain an upright posture. Engage your core, chest, and arm muscles, ensuring a firm contraction with each swing. Position your lightly clenched fists close to your jawline. With control, slowly punch in front and return to the start position, then switch to the other arm. Alternate and repeat twenty times.

Punch Down

Maintain an upright posture. Engage your core, chest, and arm muscles, ensuring a firm contraction with each swing. Bend your arms and make a fist. With control, slowly punch down and return to the start position, then switch to the other arm. Alternate and repeat twenty times.

Overhead Punches

With control, slowly punch above your head with one arm. Return to the start position, then switch to the other arm. Alternate and repeat twenty times on each side.

Upper Cuts

Sit up with your back straight and keep your feet flat on the floor. Place your hands close to your sides, forming two clenched fists facing you. Bend your elbows, pulling your fists in closer to your body. Punch each fist in an upward motion. Aim to stop the punch around chin level. Minimize unnecessary movement in the upper body. Encourage controlled breathing, exhaling with each punch. As mentioned above, controlled motion to avoid punching yourself in the face. (Real story and experience.)

Alternate between your right and left hand for each punch—repeat twenty times.

Start with a slow and controlled pace, then gradually increase speed as comfortable.

Front Punches

Maintain an upright posture. Engage your core, chest, and arm muscles, ensuring a firm contraction with each swing. Position your lightly clenched fists close to your jawline. With control, slowly punch in front and return to the start position, then switch to the other arm. Alternate and repeat twenty times.

Side Reach

Sit with your back straight and core engaged. Keep both feet flat on the floor. Knees hip-width apart.

Extend the left hand above the head, creating a shape resembling a spoon or a lengthened "C."

Hold the right side of the seat if you need to. Keep your torse engaged; don't let it collapse. Reach with your right arm to the opposite side. Alternate and repeat five to eight times on each side.

Stand Up Flow

Keep your feet flat on the floor, shoulder-width apart, and underneath your hips. Keep your back and neck straight, with your chest slightly forward. Lean forward and slightly shift your weight to the front of your feet. Slowly stand up. Try not to support any weight with your hands. Take a full breath, and tighten your core and abdominal muscles to control your lowering as much as possible. Lower yourself to the chair with control. Repeat six to ten times.

DAY 18

Front Reach

Now energetically, keep reaching to the front, slightly angling at the opposite side. Keep alternating and counting a total of twenty moves.

Sumo Chair Get Up

The feet are wider than the hips, and the toes point out slightly. Place your arms in front of you on the chair, lean slightly forward, and lift yourself, but don't fully stand up. Feel your feet firmly on the floor. Don't place the weight onto your hands—the thigh muscles are holding the weight. If you want to make it harder, remove the hands from the chair. Thighs are parallel to the floor. Repeat ten times.

Torso Twist

Put your arms behind your head and keep your elbows wide. Feel your abdominals engaged, gently twist, return to the center, and turn on another side. Alternate and repeat ten to fourteen times.

Front Punches

Keep your abdominals engaged. Bend your arms up so your wrists are by your shoulders. With control, slowly punch in front of, up, and across your body with one arm while slightly rotating your torso in the same direction. Return to the start position, then switch to the other arm. Alternate and repeat twenty times.

Extended Leg Circles

Sit up straight and lean back into the back of the chair. Kick the leg out (lifted). Pull your leg toward your chest and lean forward to meet your knee. Repeat five to eight times for each leg.

DAY 19

Heel Raises

Sit with your back straight. Ensure that both your feet are straight and the toes are facing forward. The alignment is important.

Lift your heel. Repeat each leg ten times before switching to the opposite side.

Toe Lifts

Sit with your back straight. Ensure that both your feet are straight and the toes are facing forward. The alignment is important.

Lift your toes. Repeat each leg ten times before switching to the opposite side.

Knee Extension with a Twist

Extend the leg, think of tensing the thigh muscle, release, and lower. Work on the same leg and repeat the movement eight to ten times before switching to the other side.

Stand Up Flow

Keep your feet flat on the floor, shoulder-width apart, and underneath your hips. Keep your back and neck straight, with your chest slightly forward. Lean forward and slightly shift your weight to the front of your feet. Slowly stand up. Try not to support any weight with your hands. Take a full breath, and tighten your core and abdominal muscles to control your lowering as much as possible. Lower yourself to the chair with control. Repeat six to ten times.

Elbow to Knee

Keep feet flat on the floor and shoulders rolled back. Feel your abs engaged. Place your hands behind your head, elbows pointing out to the sides. Lift your right knee toward your chest while simultaneously bringing the left elbow toward your right knee. Return to the starting position with control. Repeat on the opposite side. Alternate and repeat eight to ten times.

Seated Jacks

Move closer to the front of the chair with arms at your sides. In a harmonious motion, lift your arms overhead, fingertips gently meeting, with palms turned outward. Simultaneously, extend both legs out as your arms ascend. Bring both legs back to the center as your arms land. Repeat eight to ten times.

If extending both legs and arms simultaneously is too challenging, try this version instead.

Observe your breathing and body. Do it at a pace that suits you.

Try not to hold your breath.

Skip Rope

Rope skipping—imitate rope skipping using an imaginary rope.

Repeat thirty times.

DAY 20

Arms' Push Back

Sit closer to the edge of the chair. Lean 45 degrees forward and lift your arms with palms facing down. Take them back by lowering them and raising them behind your back as if you were making airplane arms. Repeat the movement ten to twelve times.

Marching on the Spot

March on the spot, counting a total of 30 steps.

Lateral and Front Arm Raises

Ensure your back is straight. Engage your abs. Place your arms down by your sides. Slowly lift them with weight or without parallel to the ground at shoulder level. Slowly lower them down. Lift them in front of you—shoulder level and lower them down. Control the movement; don't swing your arms. Repeat eight to ten times. You can add weights.

Hot Feet and Bicep Curl

Sit with your knees slightly apart and elbows next to your body. Start quickly running on the spot—as if the ground would feel hot, lightly tap your soles, and then incorporate a bicep curl.

Keep elbows bent at your side, turn your palms up, extend both your arms, and curl. Repeat twelve to fifteen times.

Shoulder Shrugs

Exhale and raise your shoulders slowly without bending your elbows, as if you're shrugging. At the same time, lift your heels. Keep your hands perpendicular to the floor throughout the exercise. Repeat the process in three sets of eight to twelve repetitions. As your shoulders strengthen with time, you can increase repetitions.

Step and Press

Keep your back straight, and keep the elbows bent with your palm facing out. Make a 90-degree angle on both sides (cactus arms). Press it up, and at the same time, step one foot to the side and keep your knee slightly bent. Pull your arms back and step the leg back to the center. Alternate and repeat twenty times.

Torso Twist

Put your arms in front of your chest. Imagine that you're holding a ball or weight unless you're holding it. Don't press elbows to your sides; leave some space between them. Feel your abdominals engaged, gently twist, return to the center, and turn on another side. Alternate and repeat eighteen to twenty times.

Extended Leg Circles

Sit up straight and lean back into the back of the chair. Kick the leg out (lifted). Pull your leg toward your chest and lean forward to meet your knee. Repeat five to eight times for each leg.

High Knee Pull Down

Put your arms above your head and pull them down, lifting the knee toward your chest. Lift your arms up again, and on the way down, lift an opposite knee. Repeat twenty times in total.

DAY 21

Leg and Arm Lift

Bend your arms and keep them close to your body. It's similar to a marching move. Instead of alternating, you work the same leg. The arm goes up, and the opposite knee goes toward your chest. Lift your left knee with the right arm. Repeat ten times for each leg.

Seated Jacks

Move closer to the front of the chair with arms at your sides. In a harmonious motion, lift your arms overhead, fingertips gently meeting, with palms turned outward. Simultaneously, extend both legs out as your arms ascend. Bring both legs back to the center as your arms land. Repeat eight to ten times.

If extending both legs and arms simultaneously is too challenging, try this version instead.

Observe your breathing and body. Do it at a pace that suits you.

Try not to hold your breath.

Overhead Press with a Twist

Keep the arms next to you with your palms facing in. Pull the elbows up; the shoulders are in line; the neck is nice and tall. Flip the arms over and reach above your head.

Reverse on your way back—pull elbows down (cactus arms), flip the hands over, and lower them to your side. Repeat ten to twelve times. You can use weights if you want.

Chair Mountain Climbers Variation

Lean back at a 45-degree angle. Brace yourself on the chair and bring your bottom right to the very front of it. Extend your legs out and get one knee to the chest as best as you possibly can. Maintain a 45-degree position with your upper body. Don't turn this into a crunch. Keep your torso straight, and only your knees are coming toward your chest. Alternate and repeat twenty to twenty-four times.

Back Rows

Sit up straight. Bend forward at 45 degree. Keep your arms straight next to your sides with knuckles facing outward. Raise your arms by sticking your elbows out. Repeat eight to ten times.

Step and Press

Keep your back straight, and keep the elbows bent with your palm facing out. Make a 90-degree angle on both sides (cactus arms). Press it up, and at the same time, step one foot to the side and keep your knee slightly bent. Pull your arms back and step the leg back to the center. Alternate and repeat twenty times. You can use weights.

Dumbbell Curl and Kick

Feet hip apart. Kick the right leg out and bring it back. Kick the left leg out and get it back. Hold your arm with a dumbbell with your palm facing upward. If you're not using weight, imagine that you're holding it up. Slowly curl the weight up (or just your arm) by bending your elbow,

keeping your elbow close to your body. Then, slowly lower the weight to the starting position. Now add the kick—curl both arms and right-left kick and keep alternating legs and coordinating with a bicep curl movement. Repeat twenty times.

DAY 22

Seated Side Step Over

Lift your right knee and step over the imaginary object on the floor. Lift the leg and step over it. Bring it back by stepping over back. Repeat for eight to twelve repetitions before switching to the opposite leg.

Kick and Clap

Extend one leg forward with a controlled kick, clapping your hands at shoulder height. Focus on utilizing your thigh muscles and ensuring a smooth, deliberate motion. Engage your core and kick with force, maintaining a consistent pace. Alternate legs and repeat the sequence twenty to twenty-four times.

Tap and Reach

Extend one arm diagonally as you stretch the leg on the same side in the opposite direction. Reach your fingertips toward the ceiling, lengthening the arm while stretching the leg. Focus on executing smooth, controlled movements, aiming to create a straight line from your fingertips to your toes. Alternate legs and repeat the sequence twenty to twenty-four times.

Elbow to Knee

Keep feet flat on the floor and shoulders rolled back. Feel your abs engaged. Place your hands behind your head, elbows pointing out to the sides. Lift your right knee toward your chest while simultaneously bringing the left elbow toward your right knee. Return to the starting position with control. Repeat on the opposite side. Alternate and repeat eight to ten times.

Skip Rope

Rope skipping—imitate rope skipping using an imaginary rope.

Repeat thirty times.

Step and Press

Keep your back straight, and keep the elbows bent with your palm facing out. Make a 90-degree angle on both sides (cactus arms). Press it up, and at the same time, step one foot to the side and keep your knee slightly bent. Pull your arms back and step the leg back to the center. Alternate and repeat twenty times.

DAY 23

Elegant Kick

Sit up with the back straight.

Keep both your arms straight parallel to the floor at the shoulder level. Kick your left leg out slightly, pointing to the opposite corner, and then bring it back, but keep the arms at your side. Feel your core engaged. Alternate and continue for sixteen to twenty kicks.

Front Reach

Now energetically, keep reaching to the front, slightly angling at the opposite side. Keep alternating and counting a total of twenty moves.

Front Punches

Keep your abdominals engaged. Bend your arms up so your wrists are by your shoulders. With control, slowly punch in front of, up, and across your body with one arm while slightly rotating your torso in the same direction. Return to the start position, then switch to the other arm. Alternate and repeat twenty times.

Overhead Punches

Bend your arms, and with control, slowly punch above your head with one arm. Fully straighten it, or as much as you can, and bring it down. Switch to the other arm. Alternate and repeat twenty times.

Torso Twist

Put your arms behind your head and keep your elbows wide. Feel your abdominals engaged, gently twist, return to the center, and turn on another side. Alternate and repeat ten to fourteen times.

Side Raise and Knee Raise

Keep both legs on the floor with knees bent at a 90-degree angle. Bend your elbows and lift them parallel to the floor at shoulder height. Simultaneously, lift one knee up. Bring the elbows and the knee back down. Repeat with the opposite knee—lift the elbows up with the opposite knee. Alternate and repeat twenty times. You can use weights for this movement.

Stand Up Flow

Keep your feet flat on the floor, shoulder-width apart, and underneath your hips. Keep your back and neck straight, with your chest slightly forward. Lean forward and slightly shift your weight to the front of your feet. Slowly stand up. Try not to support any weight with your hands. Take a full breath, and tighten your core and abdominal muscles to control your lowering as much as possible. Lower yourself to the chair with control. Repeat six to ten times.

Seated Shoulder Press

You can use weights if you want to, as this depends on your physical abilities. Using your body weight is also great for the workout. Engage the core muscles.

Begin with both elbows extended to the sides under the shoulders, chest lifted. Face forward with palms turned outward. Extend the arms upward, reaching above the head until fully extended or to a comfortable range. Avoid touching the hands together and keep both arms parallel. Gradually lower the hands to the starting position and maintain spread elbows. Avoid tucking the elbows toward the body's center; extend them outward until a gentle pinching sensation (not painful) is felt at the shoulder blades' top. Repeat eight to ten times.

DAY 24

Kick and Toe Touch

Take a short break if you need to. Keep the arms behind your head. Ensure you're not putting all the arm's weight and forcing your neck down. Keep your back straight and core engaged. Arms behind the head. Lift the leg and extend the opposite arm, trying to reach the toes of the opposite leg while the other arm stays behind the head. Alternate and repeat twelve to fourteen times.

Bicycle Curls

Lean back into the chair and grab the edges of the chair. Extend one leg out and pull the knee back to your chest. Think if you're peddling the bicycle. Repeat on one side six to eight times. Switch to the opposite side. Now reverse—start with one leg peddling in the opposite direction. Switch sides and repeat six to eight times.

Flutter Kicks

Lean back into the chair with your spine straight. Fully extend your legs, hold the chair's edges, lift both legs.

Single March with a Twist

Lean back into the chair with your back straight; don't round your back. Move the bottom toward the edge of the chair. You can hold the edges of the chair with your arms. Core engaged. Do single marches by lifting your knee as high as you can. Alternate and repeat ten to fourteen times.

If you're feeling brave and strong, lift both knees simultaneously. Repeat six to eight times.

and flutter. Kick your legs up and down. Repeat twenty times.

DAY 25

Modify Chair Squat

Start with your knees shoulder-width apart. Lean forward and lift your hips off the chair. If needed, you can hold the chair's edges for support as you safely return to the seated position. Alternatively, place your arms on your knees, but avoid leaning into them. Engage your glutes and hamstrings to assist in lifting your hips. Repeat this movement ten times.

Straight Leg Raise Twist

Position yourself at the front of the chair. Extend your right leg while ensuring your left foot stays grounded. Cross your arms over your chest and engage your abdominal muscles. Rotate your torso to the right, lifting your right leg.

Squeeze your knees together and return to the starting position.

Switch sides and repeat. Alternate and repeat sixteen to twenty repetitions.

Seated Jacks with Straight Arms

Put the palms together with straight arms in front of you. Hold your knees together. Move closer to the front of the chair if you need to. Open your arms to the sides and step the right foot out to the sides. Open your hips as much as you can. Arms are returning to the middle, the same as the right foot. Alternate and repeat a total of twenty times.

Lateral and Front Arm Raises

Ensure your back is straight. Engage your abs. Place your arms down by your sides. Slowly lift them with weight or without parallel to the ground at shoulder level. Slowly lower them down. Lift them in front of you—shoulder level and lower them down. Control the movement; don't swing your arms. Repeat eight to ten times. You can add weights.

Seat Hollow body

Come to the front of the chair, and with your back straight, raise your arms. Lean back at about a 45-degree angle. You should feel a contraction in your abdominals. If it feels too much with your hands over your head, cross the arms on your chest and hold. Focus on your abs. Maintain the back straight and keep leaning back.

Slowly count to 30. Take a few breaths, rest, and repeat it.

Elbow to Knee

Keep feet flat on the floor and shoulders rolled back. Feel your abs engaged. Place your hands behind your head, elbows pointing out to the sides. Lift your right knee toward your chest while simultaneously bringing the left elbow toward your right knee. Return to the starting position with control. Repeat on the opposite side. Alternate and repeat eight to ten times.

Seated Jacks

Move closer to the front of the chair with arms at your sides. In a harmonious motion, lift your arms overhead, fingertips gently meeting, with palms turned outward. Simultaneously, extend both legs out as your arms ascend. Bring both legs back to the center as your arms land. Repeat eight to ten times.

If extending both legs and arms simultaneously is too challenging, try this version instead.

Observe your breathing and body. Do it at a pace that suits you.

Try not to hold your breath.

Skater Switch

Shift to the front of your chair.

Bend your right knee while extending your left leg to the opposite side.

Keep your toes pointed.

Start extending your arms. Lean forward and attempt to reach the inside of your right foot with your left arm. Swiftly switch and repeat the movement with the right arm and the left foot. The back is straight. Alternate sides and repeat twenty-five to thirty times.

DAY 26

Hips Opener

Open both arms and hips to sides simultaneously. Repeat five to eight times.

Leg and Opposite Arm Raise

Inhale and raise the right leg and left arm. Hold for a few breaths.

Feel how your leg is activated. Lower the leg or bend through the knee if it's too challenging. Release to the ground after a couple of breaths. Repeat two to three times for each side.

Chair Squats

Stand at the back of the chair, holding onto the sides of the chair if help with balance is needed. Inhale, stand tall, grounding down into the soles of the feet, extending the spine upward. Exhale and sit weight back into heels. If you need a bigger challenge—your toes can be lifted to exaggerate the weight in the heels. Lower belly pulled in. The knees should be positioned behind the toes. Keep length in the spine and the back of the neck. Hold for three breaths. Repeat three times.

Shoulder Stretch

Bring your hands behind the head. Pull your elbows back as much as possible; imagine your shoulder blades having to keep a pencil between them. And then slowly move your elbows forward, trying to touch each other. Repeat the movement three to five times.

Lateral Arm Raises

Raise your arms parallel to the ground and at shoulder height, and lower them back to your sides. Feel your abdominal wall engaged, and don't hinge in the shoulders. Repeat the movement eight to ten times.

Plank Pose with Chair

Place your hands on the seat of the chair. Stack shoulders over hands, walk your feet back, hip-distance apart. Depending on your body's abilities, walk your feet as far as you feel comfortable. You can be on your toes or feet flat, core engaged. Observe your shoulders being stacked over your wrists. Keep your spine straight. Long line from shoulders to feet. Hold five long, deep breaths or less.

DAY 27

Elegant Kick

Sit up with the back straight.

Keep both your arms straight parallel to the floor at the shoulder level. Kick your left leg out slightly, pointing to the opposite corner, and then bring it back, but keep the arms at your side. Feel your core engaged. Alternate and continue for sixteen to twenty kicks.

Knee to Nose

Begin by standing tall and upright, squarely facing the chair seat. Place your hands on the chair. Glide your right leg behind you to its fullest extent. As you exhale, draw the right knee toward your nose, curving it inward. Inhale again, send the leg back by extending it, creating length, and then exhale to bring the knee toward your nose again. Repeat this fluid sequence a total of six to ten times on one side. Mirror the sequence on the opposite side, maintaining your focus and intention throughout.

One Leg Backlit

Keep your hands on the back of the chair. Stand tall. Bring your weight to the right foot. Extend the left leg back and lift off the ground. The toes of both feet are pointing forward. Move back and forth six to ten times. Repeat with the opposite leg. Repeat twice on each side.

Chair Pose Above Chair

Maintain an upright posture and lift your arms above your head while exhaling deeply. Inhale and move into a chair pose, gently raising yourself to your feet above the chair. Exhale and return to a seated position, arms still extended overhead. Inhale again and resume the chair pose. Repeat this sequence six times to ten times.

Step and Press

Keep your back straight, and keep the elbows bent with your palm facing out. Make a 90-degree angle on both sides (cactus arms). Press it up, and at the same time, step one foot to the side and keep your knee slightly bent. Pull your arms back and step the leg back to the center. Alternate and repeat twenty times

DAY 28

Shoulder Rolls

Start by bringing your shoulder to your ears. Slowly and gently roll them back and then forward.

Repeat ten times.

Forward Fold

On the inhale, raise your arms up and gently stretch. On the exhale, take the arms toward your feet, with the torso resting on the thighs and chin close to the knees. Feel a stretch across your shoulders and back. To release, inhale, look up first, then raise your arms before returning to sit. Remain in the pose for two breaths or till you feel comfortable.

Side Stretches

Raise your arms overhead. Extend away from the floor, maintaining open elbows. Inhale gently, drawing your shoulder blades slightly back. Engage your core and bend to the right from your torso. Exhale and switch sides. Alternate and repeat eight to ten times.

Hamstring Stretch

Sit closer to the front of the chair. Extend one leg in front of you, pulling the toes toward you. Lean as far as you can. Feel the hamstring stretch. Remain for two to three breaths. Switch the legs.

Seated Figure Four or Pigeon Pose

Put your right ankle over the left knee or on the left shin. With your back straight, lean forward and remain for a few breaths, feeling the stretch in your hip. Repeat on the other side.

Upper Body Twist

Engage your core. Keep the chin slightly tucked in. Cross your arms on your chest and twist to the right. Return to the center and then twist to the left. Alternate and repeat six to eight times.

Cat-Cow Position

Place your arms on your knees. As you inhale, expand your chest, allowing your head and chin to tilt slightly back. On the exhale, round your spine by curling your chest inward. Ensure your shoulders are relaxed, and be aware of the space between your shoulders and earlobes.

Practice coordinating your breath with the movement, moving at a comfortable pace. Repeat five to eight times.

Back Stretch

Move closer to the edge of the chair. Put your palms on your lower back and pull your elbows and shoulders back. Feel your ribcage coming forward. Remain in the position for about thirty seconds.

Conclusion

*It is exercise alone that supports the spirits,
and keeps the mind in vigor.*

— Marcus Tullius Cicero

Who would have thought that a chair could be a starting block and the finish line in the grand marathon of life, where every sprint, stumble, and snack break count?

This book has sought to guide you on your journey to physical wellness—from finding your why and starting with the combination of healthy eating and exercising to staying motivated. It should be noted in closing that this journey you are on is ever-evolving, and there is no end point, per se.

I've learned that wellness isn't a destination; it's a constantly changing landscape. It's like playing a game of tag with your former self—just when you think you've caught up, there's another version of you, slightly healthier, waving from the horizon.

So, to you, dear reader, embarking on this *chair-ful* journey to a fitter self, remember: it's a path strewn with laughter, the occasional tear, and maybe a few too many protein bars. One day, you'll look back at this version of yourself and chuckle at the memory of thinking, "How hard can exercising with a chair be?"

Embrace the journey, the chair, and maybe even the occasional indulgence. After all, what's life without a little extra seasoning? Here's to finding your balance—both on the chair and in life.

Take a seat, and happy exercising!

You Could Be Key to Someone Else's Yoga Journey

Thank you so much for your support. No matter what might hold us back from standing yoga, we can still access its astounding potential... And with your help, I can make sure that the message reaches even more people.

Transform Your Movement:
Discover our Exclusive Joint & Ankle Sequences!

Scan QR code or go on

http://chairexercises.littlegeckopublishing.com

Elevate your mobility and ease discomfort with our expertly designed sequences. Perfect for enhancing flexibility, reducing pain, or adding mindfulness to your day, these sequences are the ultimate upgrade to your wellness routine. Start feeling the difference today!

References

Admin-Calimobility. (2023, April 13). 21 Chair Exercises for Seniors: Complete visual guide. California Mobility. https://californiamobility. com/21-chair-exercises-for-seniors-visual-guide/.

Ascm-Cep, L. W. M. (2022, October 1). 11 chair exercises for seniors. Verywell Fit. https://www.verywellfit.com/chair-exercises-for-seniors-4161267.

A-Z Quotes. (n.d.). *Marcus Tullius Cicero quote*. https://www.azquotes. com/quote/566618.

BrainyQuote. (n.d.). *Friedrich Nietzsche quotes*. https://www. brainyquote.com/quotes/friedrich_nietzsche_103819.

Callahan, A., Leonard, H., & Powell, T. (2020). *Nutrition in adults*. Open Oregon Educational Resources. https://openoregon.pressbooks. pub/nutritionscience/chapter/11f-older-adults/.

Carter, C. (2012, January 2). *Please quit your diet, now*. Greater Good. https://greatergood.berkeley.edu/article/item/Quit_Diet_Now.

Centers for Disease Control and Prevention. (2019). *How much physical activity do older adults need?* https://www.cdc.gov/physicalactivity/ basics/older_adults/index.htm.

Centers for Disease Control and Prevention. (2022, September 19). *Losing weight*. https://www.cdc.gov/healthyweight/losing_weight/index.html.

Coratella, G., Tornatore, G., Longo, S., Esposito, F., & Cè, E. (2020). *An electromyographic analysis of lateral raise variations and frontal raise in competitive bodybuilders. International Journal of Environmental Research and Public Health, 17*(17) , 6015. https://doi.org/10.3390/ ijerph17176015.

Cscs, I. L. M. (2018, September 28). Seated Flexibility, Cardio, & Strength Workout. EatingWell. https://www.eatingwell.com/article/290859/seated-flexibility-cardio-strength-workout/.

Dattani, S., Ortiz-Ospina, E., Ritchie, H., Rodés-Guirao, L., & Roser, M. (2023). *Life expectancy*. Our World in Data. https://ourworldindata.org/life-expectancy.

Fitness Expo. (n.d.). How to lose weight while sitting at the office. https://www.fitnessexpostores.com/how-to-lose-weight-while-sitting-at-the-office/.

Greatist. (n.d.). Chair exercises.

 https://greatist.com/fitness/chair-exercises#sit-to-stands.

Goodreads. (n.d.). *A quote by Edward Stanley*. https://www.goodreads.com/quotes/173133-those-who-think-they-have-not-time-for-bodily-exercise.

Greenberg, M. (2013, May 21). *The best quotes on healthy living*. Psychology Today. https://www.psychologytoday.com/intl/blog/the-mindful-self-express/201305/the-best-quotes-healthy-living.

King, A. C. (2001). Interventions to promote physical activity by older adults. The Journals of Gerontology: Series A, 56(Supplement 2) , 36–46. https://doi.org/10.1093/gerona/56.suppl_2.36.

Laird, E., Rasmussen, C. L., Kenny, R. A., & Herring, M. P. (2023). Physical activity dose and depression in a cohort of older adults in the Irish Longitudinal Study on Ageing. *JAMA Network*, 6(7). https://doi.org/10.1001/jamanetworkopen.2023.22489.

Lalanne, J. (n.d.). *Quotes — Jack Lalanne*. Jack Lalanne. https://jacklalanne.com/quotes/.

Louw, S., Makwela, S., Manas, L., Meyer, L., Terblanche, D., & Brink, Y. (2017). Effectiveness of exercise in office workers with neck pain: A systematic review and meta-analysis. *South African Journal of Physiotherapy*, 73(1). https://doi.org/10.4102/sajp.v73i1.392.

Mann, T., Tomiyama, A. J., Westling, E., Lew, A.-M., Samuels, B., & Chatman, J. (2007). Medicare's search for effective obesity treatments: Diets are not the answer. *American Psychologist, 62*(3) , 220–233. https://doi.org/10.1037/0003-066x.62.3.220.

Mayo Clinic. (2023, September 21). *How do exercise and arthritis fit together?* https://www.mayoclinic.org/diseases-conditions/arthritis/in-depth/arthritis/art-20047971.

National Health Service. (2021, November 4). *Understanding calories.* https://www.nhs.uk/live-well/healthy-weight/managing-your-weight/understanding-calories/.

O'Toole, G. O. (2021, August 24). *How old would you be if you didn't know how old you are?* Quote Investigator. https://quoteinvestigator.com/2021/08/24/how-old/.

Picorelli, A. M. A., Pereira, L. S. M., Pereira, D. S., Felício, D., & Sherrington, C. (2014). Adherence to exercise programs for older people is influenced by program characteristics and personal factors: a systematic review. *Journal of Physiotherapy, 60*(3) , 151–156. https://doi.org/10.1016/j.jphys.2014.06.012.

Quote Investigator. (2019, April 18). *Take the first step in faith.* https://quoteinvestigator.com/2019/04/18/staircase/.

Seated exercise. (n.d.). https://www.active-charnwood.org/seated-exercise.

Slater, D. (2020, May 10). Lower and upper limb exercises. Keheren Therapy. https://www.keherentherapy.co.uk/chair-exercises-seniors/.

Smith, J. (2021, April 10). 5 Exercise Myths for People 55 and Older. Impact Physical Therapy. https://impactpthillsboro.com/5-exercise-myths-for-people-55-and-older/.

Smith, J. (2013, May 6). 6 seated moves that work your whole body. Shape. https://www.shape.com/fitness/workouts/6-seated-moves-work-your-whole-body.

Times of India. (n.d.). Burn the FUPA: 5 seated chair poses to get rid of lower belly fat. https://timesofindia.indiatimes.com/life-style/health-fitness/weight-loss/burn-the-fupa-5-seated-chair-poses-to-get-rid-of-lower-belly-fat/photostory/95213618.cms?picid=95213633.

U.S. Department of Health and Human Services. (2018). *Physical activity guidelines for Americans 2nd edition* (p. 32). https://health.gov/sites/default/files/2019-09/Physical_Activity_Guidelines_2nd_edition.pdf#page=32.

United Nations, Department of Economic and Social Affairs, Population Division (2022). *World Population Prospects 2022, Online Edition.* https://population.un.org/wpp/Download/Standard/Population/.

USDA. (2020). *Dietary guidelines for Americans 2020-2025.* https://www.dietaryguidelines.gov/sites/default/files/2021-03/Dietary_Guidelines_for_Americans-2020-2025.pdf.

Vive Health. (n.d.). 22 Chair exercises for Seniors & How to get started. https://www.vivehealth.com/blogs/resources/chair-exercises-for-seniors.

Website, N. (2022b, June 13). Sitting exercises. nhs.uk. https://www.nhs.uk/live-well/exercise/strength-and-flexibility-exercises/sitting-exercises/.

Wilson, C. H. (1927). [Newspaper]. Sermon.

World Health Organization. (2018). *Typhoid vaccines: WHO position paper, March 2018 — Recommendations. Vaccine, 37*(2). https://doi.org/10.1016/j.vaccine.2018.04.022.

World Health Organization. (2020, December 9). *The top 10 causes of death.* https://www.who.int/news-.

Made in the USA
Columbia, SC
14 November 2024

46529420R00070